Fatigue

THE MOST COMMON COMPLAINTS SERIES

Headache
Egilius L. H. Spierings

Confusion
Karl E. Misulis and Terri Edwards-Lee

Neck Complaints
Michael Ronthal

Chest Pain
Richard C. Becker

Gait Disorders
Michael Ronthal

Smell and Taste Complaints
Christopher H. Hawkes

Fatigue

Lauren B. Krupp, MD

Professor of Neurology
State University of New York at Stony Brook
Stony Brook, New York

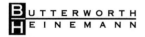

An Imprint of Elsevier Science

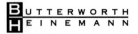

An Imprint of Elsevier Science

The Curtis Center
Independence Square West
Philadelphia, PA 19106

FATIGUE   ISBN 0-7506-7038-X

Copyright 2003, Elsevier Science (USA).

Notice

Medicine is an ever-changing field. Standard safety precautions must be followed but as new research and clinical experience broaden our knowledge, changes in treatment and drug therapy may become necessary or appropriate. Readers are advised to check the most current product information provided by the manufacturer of each drug to be administered to verify the recommended dose, the method and duration of administration, and contraindications. It is the responsibility of the treating physician, relying on experience and knowledge of the patient, to determine dosages and the best treatment for each individual patient. Neither the Publisher nor the author assumes any liability for any injury and/or damage to persons or property arising from this publication.

Every effort has been made to ensure that the drug dosage schedules within this text are accurate and conform to standards accepted at time of publication. However, as treatment recommendations vary in the light of continuing research and clinical experience, the reader is advised to verify drug dosage schedules herein with information found on product information sheets. This is especially true in cases of new or infrequently used drugs.

Recognizing the importance of preserving what has been written, Elsevier Science prints its books on acid-free paper whenever possible.

The Publisher

First Edition

Library of Congress Cataloging-in-Publication Data

Krupp, Lauren B.
    Fatigue / Lauren B. Krupp.– 1st ed.
      p. ; cm. – (The most common complaints series)
    Includes bibliographical references and index.
    ISBN 0-7506-7038-x
      1. Fatigue. I. Title. II. Series.
      [DNLM: 1. Fatigue–physiopathology. WB 146 K94f 2003]
    RB150.F37K78 2003
    612′.042–de21

                                                                                    2002036113

British Library Cataloguing-in-Publication Data
A catalogue record for this book is available from the British Library.

The publisher offers special discounts on bulk orders of this book.
For information, please contact:

Manager of Special Sales
Elsevier Science
625 Walnut Street
Philadelphia, PA 19106
Tel: 215-238-7800
Fax: 215-238-8483

For information on all
Elsevier Health Sciences
publications available,
contact our World Wide Web
home page at:
www.elsevierhealth.com

Editor: Susan F. Pioli
Editorial Assistant: Joan Ryan
Production Editor: Mary Stermel

10 9 8 7 6 5 4 3 2 1

Printed in the United States of America

This book is dedicated to individuals with a diagnosis of multiple sclerosis, their family, and their friends.

This book is dedicated to individuals with a diagnosis of multiple sclerosis, their family, and their friends.

Contents

Acknowledgments   ix

1. Introduction   1

Part One: Concepts in Fatigue Management

2. Fatigue Definitions and Epidemiology   9
3. Measurement of Fatigue   29
4. Fatigue Covariables   45
5. Fatigue Pathophysiology   59
6. The Fatigue Workup   79

Part Two: Fatigue in Specific Disorders

7. Multiple Sclerosis–Related Fatigue   91

8. Fatigue in Postpolio Syndrome   113
9. Parkinson's Disease   123
10. Cancer-Related Fatigue   131
11. Postoperative Fatigue   145
12. Systemic Lupus Erythematosus   157
13. Lyme Disease   169
14. HIV–Related Fatigue   177
15. Chronic Fatigue Syndrome   185
16. Chronic Obstructive Pulmonary Disease   199

Part Three: Fatigue Management

17. Treatment Approaches   207
18. Conclusions   229

Index   233

Acknowledgments

Thank you to Alexa, Gina, and my family for making this book possible. I am grateful to Harold Schombert for his assistance with this book, and for the support provided by an educational grant from Cephalon.

CHAPTER ONE

Introduction

Ask patients or physicians to describe what *fatigue* is, and you will probably get a wide variety of definitions and descriptions that range from tiredness, sleepiness, and weakness to exhaustion and languor. The truth is fatigue can be an extremely amorphous concept, and the understanding of fatigue can vary tremendously depending on the type of patient and the background of the provider.

The fact that there are so many different concepts of fatigue makes it a difficult symptom to define, assess, and treat. This is unfortunate because fatigue is one of the most frequent symptoms in all of medicine. Most commonly understood as an overwhelming sense of tiredness that is out of proportion to "normal" tiredness, fatigue is associated with a range of conditions, including cancer, infectious disorders, autoimmune conditions such as multiple sclerosis, and sequelae from acute events such as stroke or postoperative states (Box 1-1). In some illnesses, such as multiple sclerosis, the vast majority of patients have reported fatigue at some point.[1]

Regardless of the disorder, fatigue can have a major impact on patient functioning and activities of daily living, on quality of life, on employment, and on psychological well-being.[2,3] The effects are not limited to the patient: The individual's family can suffer as well.[4] Despite the high frequency and impact of fatigue, research shows that it is given insufficient attention by health care providers and patients alike. In one study of more than 1300 cancer patients, although 58% reported being "somewhat fatigued" or "very much fatigued," only 52% of those with fatigue ever reported it to their hospital physician, and only 14% had received treatment or advice about their fatigue.[5]

The challenge to the health care provider is to identify fatigue, and once it is identified, to treat it appropriately. This challenge is not an easy one. Many healthy individuals experience fatigue at various times in their lives; studies have indicated a fatigue prevalence of approximately 20% among the general population.[6] The words used to describe

Box 1-1. Some Disorders Associated with Fatigue in which Clinical Research Has Been Performed

Autoimmune Disorders
- Multiple sclerosis
- Systemic lupus erythematosus

Malignancy
- Cancer-related anemia

Infections
- Lyme disease
- Human immunodeficiency virus (HIV) infection/AIDS
- Postpolio syndrome

Postoperative States

Sequelae from Neurologic Diseases/Injury
- Parkinson's disease
- Stroke
- Head trauma

Conditions of Unknown Cause
- Chronic fatigue syndrome

Fibromyalgia/Rheumatologic Disorders

Psychiatric Illnesses
- Major depression

Endocrine Disorders
- Thyroid disease
- Pregnancy

Cardiac and Pulmonary Disorders
- Obstructive sleep apnea and other sleep disorders
- Chronic obstructive pulmonary disease
- Deconditioning

fatigue are not exclusive to a pathologic state, making the identification of illness-related fatigue difficult. In some cases, fatigue has a clearly defined association (e.g., anemia) that responds to specific treatments. In other cases, the cause of fatigue is not evident.

Although the immune system appears to play an important role in fatigue, physiologic factors such as pain or deconditioning, and psychological factors such as depression, are strongly related to fatigue symptoms. Because much of the diagnosis of fatigue is based on the self-report of the patient, asking patients to describe their fatigue and to separate it from these other concepts is often unrealistic. Identifying fatigue clearly depends on what questions are asked, and what diagnostic criteria are used. It is often necessary to assess patients for the presence or absence of potential overlapping or confounding symptoms.

This book is a practical guide to the assessment and management of fatigue. The first section addresses the epidemiology of fatigue in various clinical populations, and the pathophysiologic mechanisms related to fatigue. The primary covariates to fatigue are discussed, including pain, mood, cognitive functioning, and sleep disorders, and practical means to diagnose fatigue in the patient with neurologic disease are reviewed. The second section of this book discusses characteristics of fatigue in individual medical disorders, such as multiple sclerosis, cancer, systemic lupus erythematosus, and chronic fatigue syndrome, and identifies a number of treatment strategies, including behavioral approaches and pharmacologic agents. This book can be used both as a guide for health care providers who are likely to encounter fatigue in their practice, as well as physicians, researchers, or other providers who are interested in having an introduction to the topic and a guide for additional inquiry. Although the book is not meant to be all-encompassing, or to represent the entirety of medical and nonmedical research on the subject of fatigue, several important scientific concepts related to fatigue and key diagnostic and treatment principles are presented to the reader. Additional reading can be found in the references cited throughout the text and at the end of each chapter.

REFERENCES

1. Freal JE, Kraft GH, Coryell JK. Symptomatic management in multiple sclerosis. Arch Phys Med Rehabil 65:135–138, 1984.
2. Hann DM, Garovoy N, Finkelstein B, et al. Fatigue and quality of life in breast cancer patients undergoing autologous stem cell transplantation: a

longitudinal comparative study. J Pain Symptom Manage 17:311–319, 1999.

3. Pawlikowska T, Chalder T, Hirsch SR, et al. Population based study of fatigue and psychological distress. BMJ 308:763–766, 1994.

4. Hamilton J, Butler L, Wagenaar H, et al. The impact and management of cancer-related fatigue on patients and families. Can Oncol Nurs J 11:192–198, 2001.

5. Stone P, Richards M, A'Hern R, Hardy J. A study to investigate the prevalence, severity and correlates of fatigue among patients with cancer in comparison with a control group of volunteers without cancer. Ann Oncol 11:561–567, 2000.

6. Loge JH, Ekeberg O, Kaasa S. Fatigue in the general Norwegian population: Normative data and associations. J Psychosom Res 45:53–65, 1998.

PART ONE

Concepts in Fatigue Management

CHAPTER TWO

Fatigue Definitions and Epidemiology

In searching the literature for a concrete definition of fatigue in medical illness, one thing quickly becomes clear. This is truly a symptom in which the answer begs the question. Even in chronic fatigue syndrome (CFS), an illness in which fatigue essentially defines the disorder, the word *fatigue* is not defined by the Centers for Disease Control and Prevention's (CDC) case definition per se; it is merely reiterated as one of the hallmark symptoms of the disease (Box 2-1).[1] Reading the CDC's case definition, it is no clearer to the average physician exactly what fatigue is.

In truth, much of the difficulty in defining fatigue stems from limitations in our vocabulary. The word *fatigue* is, at the same time, tremendously meaningful and terribly imprecise. Because it is a

---

Box 2-1. Centers for Disease Control Case Definition for Chronic Fatigue Syndrome

1. Clinically evaluated, unexplained persistent or relapsing chronic fatigue that is of new or definite onset (i.e., not lifelong), is not the result of ongoing exertion, is not substantially alleviated by rest, and results in substantial reduction in previous levels of occupational, educational, social, or personal activities.

2. The concurrent occurrence of four or more of the following symptoms. These symptoms must have persisted or recurred during 6 or more consecutive months, and must not have predated the fatigue:
   - substantial impairment in short-term memory or concentration
   - sore throat
   - tender lymph nodes
   - muscle pain
   - multijoint pain without swelling or redness
   - headaches of a new type, pattern, or severity
   - unrefreshing sleep
   - postexertional malaise lasting more than 24 hours

(Source: Centers for Disease Control. Case definition for chronic fatigue syndrome. Available at http://www.cdc.gov/ncidod/diseases/cfs/defined.html. Last accessed September 20, 2002.)

word of common usage in everyday speech, there is a danger of presupposing that we know precisely what the patient means by the word. A number of other terms are used interchangeably with fatigue, including malaise, asthenia, and weakness. The patient may also use the word fatigue to describe two different states during a single encounter.

When physicians or other health care providers hear patients say the word fatigue, it is up to the physician or health care provider to determine as accurately as possible what the patient means. Are they physically tired during the day? Are they mentally exhausted? Are they lacking in motivation? Are they having difficulty concentrating? Do they feel depressed? Do they feel tired after a full night's sleep, or have they been having sleep problems? Have they experienced an abnormal lack of performance? Is the problem confined to a specific limb or body part? Is there significant interference with the ability to perform the tasks of daily life? Is there significant physical discomfort or pain? These concepts can all mean different things, yet have all been used to describe fatigue.[2–6]

This language gap of fatigue is by no means limited to the physician-patient interaction. The term fatigue may also mean markedly different things to different specialists and subspecialists. Neurologists who are experienced with the postpolio patient will probably have a much different conception of fatigue than neurologists experienced with the multiple sclerosis (MS) patient, and this will differ still from the conception of physicians experienced with depression treatment.

A multidimensional view of fatigue has emerged from the descriptions that have been given the symptom. Fatigue incorporates a number of concepts, including:

- Decreased mental and physical endurance
- Decreased motivation
- Depletion of reserves
- Fatigability
- Inability to rise to the occasion
- Performance that is short of one's expectations (as when healthy)
- Lassitude

Unfortunately, one of the greatest challenges in defining fatigue is that there are few, if any, objective criteria that can help physicians "see" fatigue for themselves. Other than certain cases of neuromuscular fatigue that can be quantified through tests of force generation,[7] the ability to define and identify fatigue rests almost entirely in the hands of the patient's experience, and what he or she can tell us. Many physicians have gone as far as to suggest that fatigue should be considered abnormal simply when the patient says that it is.[8] Although diagnosis certainly involves more than that—in cancer-related fatigue, for example, anemia can be quantified, and in any form of fatigue, diagnostic surveys can be assessed for their reliability—the physician must always have an abiding respect for patients' reports of their symptoms.

Not nearly enough work has been done in the area of defining fatigue—a fact that is a little surprising, given that reports of fatigue in many diseases are often the rule, rather than the exception, and given that fatigue is often listed as the greatest impediment of all to a satisfactory quality of life. In one study, not only was fatigue highly frequent, it tended to be long lasting, with more than 40% of patients reporting feeling fatigued every day of the month (Fig. 2-1).[9,10]

In addition, our definitions have failed to adequately address the issue of "normal" versus abnormal, or pathologic, fatigue. When we assess the patient for fatigue, we often treat fatigue as an entity that is either present or absent. This distinction is somewhat artificial, as everyone feels fatigued at some time, and even those who experience normal fatigue may also experience pathologic fatigue.[8] It is likely that fatigue falls along a continuum, in much the same way that blood pressure does, with some patients experiencing low levels of

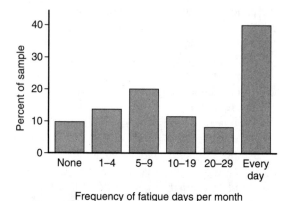

Frequency of fatigue days per month

Figure 2-1. Frequency of fatigue problems during the past 30 days for MS patients. (Reprinted with permission from Fisk JD, Pontefract A, Ritvo PG, et al. The impact of fatigue on patients with multiple sclerosis. Can J Neurol Sci 21:9–14, 1994.)

fatigue, some experiencing extremely high levels, and the remainder feeling normal levels. This is what is referred to as the *dimensional,* rather than the *categorical,* view of fatigue, and the accompanying challenge is to determine not only when fatigue is present, but when it is pathologic (Fig. 2-2).[8] In our research, one distinction that we found between healthy volunteers and individuals with

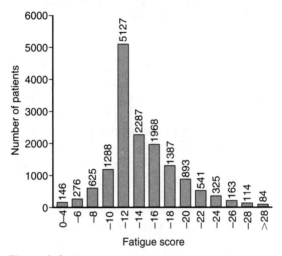

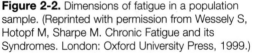

Figure 2-2. Dimensions of fatigue in a population sample. (Reprinted with permission from Wessely S, Hotopf M, Sharpe M. Chronic Fatigue and its Syndromes. London: Oxford University Press, 1999.)

MS is that, although the quality of fatigue did not differ, there was a significant inability to perform activities of daily living in the patient group. The deleterious effects of fatigue on quality of life or meeting responsibilities, therefore, may represent pathologic fatigue.[11]

FATIGUE IN THE GENERAL POPULATION

Many large-scale surveys have been conducted on the prevalence and severity of fatigue in the general population. Making generalized statements about the prevalence of fatigue by citing population-based surveys is difficult because these surveys necessarily contain the same definitional limitations of fatigue. Epidemiologic surveys can vary widely in the words used (e.g., sleepiness, tiredness, weakness) and this imprecision can yield far different survey results.

For example, one research group of CFS from England pointed to the experience in two versions of a UK National Medical Ambulatory Care Survey. In 1977, the definition of fatigue changed following the first survey to eliminate the concept of general weakness. As a result, a significant decrease in the percentage of persons with fatigue was recorded between the two surveys, without a change in the participants' actual circumstances.[8] (This lesson has implications not only for the epidemiologist but also for the physician involved in clinical care. It is important to use consistent terms and consistent instruments, if possible, throughout the course of assessment, diagnosis, intervention, and follow-up.)

Studies consistently show that fatigue is highly prevalent in the general population and in those who seek care at the primary physician level: Up to 20% of men and 25% of women in the general population "always feel tired," and this fatigue not infrequently leads to a health care provider visit. Therefore, a primary care provider is likely to encounter at least one fatigue patient every day of the week in his or her practice.[12] There is much room for improvement in management, because at least 25% of fatigue in primary care goes undiagnosed.[8]

FATIGUE IN MEDICAL POPULATIONS

Epidemiologic surveys have shown that fatigue is a major symptom and highly prevalent in a number of disorders, including CFS, systemic lupus erythematosus (SLE), epilepsy, Parkinson's disease (PD), cancer, and MS. Unfortunately, because it is a potentially nonspecific disease symptom, it often escapes physician awareness. For example, fatigue in MS has a reported frequency as high as 97%, yet is not routinely considered a hallmark symptom of the disease.[10,11,13] Meanwhile, "less frequent" symptoms of MS problems, including weakness, numbness, or bowel and bladder difficulties, are more routinely emphasized (Table 2-1).[13]

Table 2-1. Top Five Symptoms Reported by a Sample of 656 MS Patients

Symptom	No ADL Difficulty (%)	Producing ADL Difficulty (%)
Fatigue	22	56
Balance problems	24	50
Weakness/paralysis	18	45
Numbness/tingling/other sensory disturbance	39	24
Bladder problems	25	34

ADL, activities of daily living.
(Reprinted with permission from Freal JE, Kraft GH, Coryell JK. Symptomatic fatigue in multiple sclerosis. Arch Phys Med Rehabil 65:135–138, 1984.)

Perhaps because physicians caring for the MS patient until 1993 had only symptomatic therapies to offer for this chronic condition, there has been an accumulation of scientific studies in this field, which may explain why it is one of the only conditions for which a consensus definition has been reached. In 1998, the MS Council for Clinical Practice Guidelines provided a working definition of fatigue and made recommendations regarding its evaluation, measurement, and treatment (Table 2-2).[14]

Although a great degree of understanding of fatigue in neurology has taken place in the MS community, other disorders of both neurologic and non-neurologic causes are associated with fatigue. In one survey of an epilepsy population, severe

Table 2-2. The Definition of Multiple Sclerosis–Related Fatigue

Fatigue is a subjective lack of physical and/or mental energy that is perceived by the individual or caregiver to interfere with usual and desired activities.

Chronic persistent fatigue:
1. Fatigue that is present for any amount of time on 50% of the days for more than 6 weeks
2. Fatigue that limits functional activities or quality of life

Acute fatigue:
1. New or a significant increase in feelings of fatigue in the previous 6 weeks
2. Fatigue that limits functional activities or quality of life

(Source: MS Council for Clinical Practice Guidelines. Fatigue in Multiple Sclerosis. Washington, DC: Paralyzed Veterans Association, 1998.)

fatigue was reported by 44%.[15] Fatigue may stem from some pathophysiologic mechanism in epilepsy. It is also significantly related to the medications used to treat the disease, many of which have sedating properties.[15]

Fatigue is frequent in PD, with almost 60% considering it to be one of the three most disabling symptoms of the disease.[16] Fatigue may potentially be related to the neurologic changes in the brain, the difficulties in performance of motor tasks, or a side effect of PD therapies such as dopamine agonists.

Fatigue is an important complaint in SLE, and one of the most debilitating symptoms. In one study, fatigue was reported by 85.7% of 225 patients with recent onset of SLE (≤5 years).[17] During an exacerbation of SLE, fatigue is prominent and often precedes other signs of organ involvement. SLE appears to present in tandem approximately one quarter of the time with fibromyalgia, which also has a significant fatigue component.[18]

Fatigue in the form of muscle tiredness is very common in the literature on postpolio syndrome. These patients have described a feeling of tiredness using specific muscles or groups of muscles (e.g., the patient can only produce one or two forceful contractions, instead of 5 or 10). Along with pain and breathing difficulties, fatigue is a late effect of polio infection.[19]

Depending on the form of treatment that they are undergoing, virtually all cancer patients may be affected by fatigue (Table 2-3).[20,21] Studies have shown that it is more frequent than pain or anxiety,

Table 2-3. Prevalence of Fatigue in Cancer Patients by Treatment Status

Fatigue and cancer (untreated)	78%
Fatigue and chemotherapy	60%–90%
Fatigue and radiation therapy	75%–100%

(Reprinted with permission from Sobrero A, Puglisi F, Guglielmi A, et al. Fatigue: a main component of anemia symptomatology. Semin Oncol 28[suppl 8]:15–18, 2001.)

and more than twice as frequent as nausea. Unlike fatigue in so many other disorders, some aspects of cancer-related fatigue (and fatigue related to postoperative blood loss and hemodialysis) can be linked to a specific cause. For example, cancer-associated anemia is strongly associated with fatigue, and treatment with recombinant human erythropoietin, iron supplementation, or red blood cell transfusion can reduce fatigue.

The high frequency of fatigue in the postoperative patient may come as a surprise. Nearly three quarters of posthysterectomy patients experience debilitating fatigue, and more than one third reported that fatigue is the factor most likely to interfere with recovery.[22] It occurred more frequently and lasted twice as long as pain, contributed to feelings of frustration in more than half of patients, and also led to difficulties in concentration in 42%.

Anemia may also contribute to fatigue associated with human immunodeficiency virus (HIV) infection, although fatigue in the HIV patient is also caused by nutritional deficiencies, depression, and concomitant infections. In one survey of 504 ambulatory patients with acquired immunodeficiency syndrome (AIDS), fatigue was present in 85% of patients—even more than pain or sadness. The only symptom that was more prevalent was worrying.[23] Fatigue was a significant predictor of quality of life.[24]

Fatigue is a major feature of infectious conditions, both during acute illness and in some cases during chronic infection. Acute viral syndromes, active Lyme disease, and a variety of other infectious disorders are associated with malaise and fatigue. Some of the pioneering work establishing psychological correlates of persistent fatigue was completed more than 60 years ago in studies of the Asian Flu epidemic. In addition to acute infection, chronic infectious disorders including infectious mononucleosis, chronic hepatitis, and chronic Lyme disease are responsible for overwhelming fatigue.

The formalization of the disorder of CFS in 1988 and its subsequent revision in 1994 helped spur a series of investigations related to this symptom. Fatigue is the core feature of CFS and is a major criterion of the CDC definition. The other major criterion requires the exclusion of other known causes of fatigue. Nevertheless, CFS is often associated with a variety of other minor problems such as arthralgia, sleep disturbance, and myalgia.

Chronic fatigue syndrome may be confused with another disorder, post-Lyme syndrome, because the two have much overlap in terms of symptomatology. It has been estimated that 82% of patients with post-Lyme syndrome meet the criteria for CSF, and that they do not differ from each other in the presentation of fatigue.[25]

The occurrence of fatigue in any of these disorders may be highly sensitive to time and place. For example, patients who are asked about their fatigue at 8 AM are likely to give a much different answer than patients who are asked about their fatigue at 5 PM. A seasonal severity for symptoms, including fatigue, was reported in a study of nearly 1500 patients with rheumatic diseases, including osteoarthritis, rheumatoid arthritis, and fibromyalgia.[26] The greatest severity of symptoms was seen in December and January, with the lowest severity in July.

The epidemiologic surveys have done a reasonable job in examining fatigue by gender and socioeconomic status. The literature on fatigue shows a consistent preference for fatigue in women, with a ratio of approximately 1.5:1.[8] A number of reasons have been posed for this. It may be that women complain more to their care providers about symptoms that men may consider to be minor. Perhaps women experience fatigue for longer periods of time, and are thus more likely to be fatigued during any particular assessment. Women may also be subject to a greater incidence of depression, which has a strong association with fatigue.[8]

The data on fatigue and socioeconomic class are somewhat surprising, given that fatigue is often believed to be a disease of the educated and wealthy

Fatigue Definitions and Epidemiology: Key Concepts

- The word *fatigue* is used by health care providers and patients alike to refer to a number of concepts, including decreased mental and physical endurance, decreased motivation, and performance that is short of one's expectations. It is important for physicians to determine exactly what patients mean when they report feeling fatigued.

- Fatigue is the rule rather than the exception in a wide variety of disorders, including neurologic illness, cancer, CFS, chronic infectious states, and postoperative states. Therefore, its presence should be presupposed until proven otherwise.

- Fatigue likely falls along a continuum much the same way that blood pressure does, with some people having normal levels of fatigue, and others having abnormally high (or low) levels.

- Epidemiologic studies show that fatigue has a prevalence of 20% to 25% in primary care populations. Women tend to report fatigue more often than men, and those of lower socioeconomic status more often than those of higher socioeconomic status.

- Fatigue can be highly sensitive to time and place; it is important for physicians to keep in mind the time of day (e.g., morning versus early evening), the patient's degree of activity during the day, and even the seasons.

(think about the "yuppie flu" epidemic of the 1980s). In fact, the opposite is true, with lower socioeconomic classes actually having a greater incidence.[8] This conclusion makes sense, given that fatigue may be tied to depressive symptoms, which are more likely to occur among those who lack both social support and the means to attain such support.

The only remarkable factor about age and fatigue is that fatigue appears to be negligible before adolescence. Otherwise, fatigue does not appear to increase with age. Hence, if an elderly individual presents with a chief complaint of new-onset fatigue, this problem should never be attributed simply to advanced age. While little analyses have been done on the issue of race and fatigue, those that have tend to show slightly higher fatigue scores in whites than in Hispanics or African Americans, although the difference is not significant.

CONCLUSIONS

The difficulties in defining fatigue should make the health care provider no less respectful of the symptom and its impact, which is substantial according to the majority of accounts. Fatigue can be just as much a part of a patient's illness as any of the traditional "hallmark" signs or symptoms. It is true that, depending on the question asked, the incidence of fatigue could vary widely. Nevertheless, the majority of surveys, regardless of the wording used, tend to show a very high prevalence of fatigue, emphasizing that fatigue as a symptom is not to be taken lightly. Our ability to make a more accurate assessment of fatigue will improve as our understanding of the symptom increases and our terms for defining fatigue become more precise.

REFERENCES

1. Centers for Disease Control. Case definition for chronic fatigue syndrome. Available at: http://www.cdc.gov/ncidod/diseases/cfs/ defined.html. Last accessed September 20, 2002.
2. Schwid SR, Thornton CA, Pandya S, et al. Quantitative assessment of motor fatigue and strength in MS. Neurology 53:743–750, 1999.
3. Weinshenker BG, Penman M, Bass B, et al. A double-blind, randomized, crossover trial of pemoline in fatigue associated with multiple sclerosis. Neurology 42:1468–1471, 1992.
4. Iriarte J, Subira ML, de Castro P. Modalities of fatigue in multiple sclerosis: correlation with clinical and biological factors. Mult Scler 6:124–130, 2000.
5. Holley S. Cancer-related fatigue: suffering a different fatigue. Cancer Practice 8:87–95, 2000.
6. Knowles G. Survey of nurses' assessment of cancer-related fatigue. Eur J Cancer Care 9:105–113, 2000.

7. Kent-Braun JA, LeBlanc R. Quantitation of central activation failure during maximal voluntary contractions in humans. Muscle Nerve 19:861–869, 1996.

8. Wessely S, Hotopf M, Sharpe M. Chronic Fatigue and its Syndromes. London: Oxford University Press, 1999.

9. Fisk JD, Pontefract A, Ritvo PG, et al. The impact of fatigue on patients with multiple sclerosis. Can J Neurol Sci 21:9–14, 1994.

10. Vercoulen JG, Hommes OR, Swanink CM, et al. The measurement of fatigue in patients with multiple sclerosis. A multidimensional comparison with patients with chronic fatigue syndrome and healthy subjects. Arch Neurol 53:642–649, 1996.

11. Krupp LB, Alvarez LA, LaRocca NG, Scheinberg LC. Fatigue in multiple sclerosis. Arch Neurol 45:435–437, 1988.

12. Katon WJ, Buchwald DS, Simon GE, et al. Psychiatric illness in patients with chronic fatigue and those with rheumatoid arthritis. J Gen Intern Med 6:277–285, 1991.

13. Freal JE, Kraft GH, Coryell JK. Symptomatic fatigue in multiple sclerosis. Arch Phys Med Rehabil 65:138, 1984.

14. MS Council for Clinical Practice Guidelines. Fatigue in Multiple Sclerosis. Washington, DC: Paralyzed Veterans Association, 1998.

15. Ettinger AB, Weisbrot DM, Krupp LB, et al. Fatigue and depression in epilepsy. J Epilepsy 11:105;109, 1998.

16. Ziv I, Avraham M, Michaelov Y, et al. Enhanced fatigue during motor performance in patients with

Parkinson's disease. Neurology 51:1583–1586, 1998.

17. Zonana-Nacach A, Roseman JM, McGwin G, et al. Systemic lupus erythematosus in three ethnic groups, VI: factors associated with fatigue within 5 years of criteria diagnosis. Lupus 9:101–109, 2000.

18. Tench CM, McCurdie I, White PDC, D'Cruz DP. The prevalence and associations of fatigue in systemic lupus erythematosus. Rheumatology 39:1249–1254, 2000.

19. Schanke AK, Stanghelle JK. Fatigue in polio survivors. Spinal Cord 39:243–251, 2001.

20. Meek PM, Nail LM, Barsevick A, et al. Psychometric testing of fatigue instruments for use in cancer patients. Nursing Research 49:181–190, 2000.

21. Sobrero A, Puglisi F, Guglielmi A, et al. Fatigue: a main component of anemia symptomatology. Semin Oncol 28:15–18, 2001.

22. DeCherney AH, Bachmann G, Isaacson K, Gall S. Postoperative fatigue negatively impacts the daily lives of patients recovering from hysterectomy. Obstet Gynecol 99:51–57, 2002.

23. Vogel D, Rosenfeld B, Breitbart W, et al. Symptom prevalence, characteristics, and distress in AIDS outpatients. J Pain Symptom Manage 18:253–262, 1998.

24. Eller LS. Quality of life in persons living with HIV. Clin Nurs Res 10:401–423, 2001.

25. Guadino EA, Coyle PK, Krupp LB. Post-lyme syndrome and chronic fatigue syndrome. Arch Neurol 54:1372–1376, 1997.

26. Hawley DJ, Wolfe F, Lue FA, Moldofsky H. Seasonal symptom severity in patients with rheumatic diseases: a study of 1,424 patients. J Rheumatol 28:1900–1909, 2001.

Measurement of Fatigue

There are a number of approaches to measuring fatigue in the patient with medical illnesses, including self-report scales that assess the individual's perceived level of fatigue, and objective, performance-based measures that assess various neurophysiologic parameters such as muscle force generation. This chapter addresses general issues in the measurement of fatigue. As with other areas of fatigue management, measurement issues have been explored more deeply in certain disease states than in others. Issues related more specifically to various disorders will be discussed in the chapters on those diseases.

SELF-REPORT MEASURES

Self-report scales are the most widely used methods of measuring fatigue, and have been the tools employed in most clinical investigations. These scales, which all measure the patient's perceived level of fatigue, have a number of advantages that also make them useful for clinical practice. They are generally short, are widely available, are easily understandable by the patient, and require little prior learning by the physician and/or staff. The summary score can be used, or scores can be averaged

There is a wide range of self-report scales available for fatigue measurement, ranging from simple, unidimensional measures to more complex tools that assess multiple dimensions such as physical and social functioning. The simplest example of a unidimensional scale is the single-item Visual Analog Scale for Fatigue (VAS-F), a 10-cm line diagram that asks patients to assess their degree of fatigue on a scale of 0 (not at all fatigued) to 100 (fatigue as bad as can be) (Fig. 3-1).[1] The VAS-F has been used in a number of clinical evaluations of fatigue, including multiple sclerosis (MS).[1]

There are a number of other fatigue scales available of varying complexity, including the Fatigue Severity Scale (FSS)[2]; the Fatigue Impact Scale (FIS)[3]; the Modified Fatigue Impact Scale

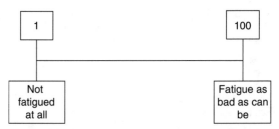

Figure 3-1. Visual Analog Scale for Fatigue, a simple assessment tool in which patients are asked to rate their level of fatigue on a scale of 0 (not at all fatigued) to 100 (fatigue as bad as can be). (Reprinted with permission from Weinshenker BG, Penman M, Bass B, et al. A double-blind, randomized crossover trial of pemoline in fatigue associated with multiple sclerosis. Neurology 42:1468–1471, 1992.)

(MFIS),[4] which along with the FSS is widely used in studies of MS; and the Fatigue Scale,[5] which attempts to distinguish physical and mental dimensions of fatigue (Table 3-1).[2–13] The scores of these scales may differ in subtle ways across different disorders. For example, it has been suggested that in the chronic fatigue syndrome (CFS) population, the Fatigue Scale focuses more on the intensity of fatigue, whereas the FSS assesses to a greater extent functional outcomes of fatigue.[14] In contrast, in studies of head trauma, the FIS may be more comprehensive than the FSS.[15]

Table 3-1. Selected Fatigue Scales Used in a Variety of Medical Conditions or Covering Disease Specific Fatigue Features

Checklist of Individual Strength (CIS)[7]
Fatigue Assessment Instrument (FAI)[9]
Fatigue Descriptive Scale (FDS)[10]
Fatigue Impact Scale (FIS)[3]
Fatigue Scale (FS)[5]
Fatigue Severity Scale (FSS)[2]
Fatigue Symptom Inventory (FSI)[12]
Medical Outcomes Survey-Short Form 36 (SF-36)[13]
Modified Fatigue Impact Scale (MFIS)[4]
Multidimensional Assessment of Fatigue (MAF)[6]
Multidimensional Fatigue Inventory (MFI)[8]
Profile of Mood States (POMS)[11]

(Sources: Krupp, 1989; Fisk, 1994; MS Council for Clinical Practice Guidelines, 1998; Chalder, 1993; Belza, 1993; Vercoulen, 1996; Smets, 1995; Schwartz, 1993; Iriarte, 1999; McNair, 1992; Hann, 2000; Ware, 1994.)

Examples of scales designed to assess multiple dimensions, including social and physical functioning, include the Multidimensional Fatigue Inventory (MFI) and the Multidimensional Assessment of Fatigue (MAF), both of which have been used in a variety of disease groups, including arthritis, cancer, CFS, and pulmonary disease.[6,8,16] Despite the advantages of assessing multiple aspects of fatigue, these measures may show less robust psychometric properties of reliability, validity, and responsiveness than unidimensional fatigue measures such as the fatigue subscale of the Profile of Mood States (POMS). This has been the case in cancer patients.[17] The fatigue subscale of the POMS is similar to the vitality subscale of the Medical Outcomes Survey Short Form 36 (SF-36), in that both are assessments of either fatigue or its inverse (i.e., vitality), contained in a larger, more comprehensive perceived health inventory.

In many cases, specific scales have been designed to assess fatigue in specific disease populations. For example, the Fatigue Descriptive Scale (FDS)[10] and the MS-Specific Fatigue Scale (MS-FS)[18] ask questions about the effects of fatigue on heat, factors that are of particular importance to the MS patient. The Fatigue Symptom Inventory (FSI) was developed primarily for cancer-related fatigue.[12] Choosing a particular fatigue measure requires an understanding of the purpose of the investigation and the specific characteristics of the patient population of interest.

The FSS is a nine-item scale that assesses disabling fatigue in various medical populations (Table 3-2).[2] The scale was developed as an improved method over the VAS-F, as it is more resistant to impulsive answering. The FSS, like many of these scales, can be scored using the sum

Table 3-2. Fatigue Severity Scale

Statement	Score
1. My motivation is lower when I am fatigued.	_____
2. Exercise brings on my fatigue.	_____
3. I am easily fatigued.	_____
4. Fatigue interferes with my physical functioning.	_____
5. Fatigue causes frequent problems for me.	_____
6. My fatigue prevents sustained physical functioning.	_____
7. Fatigue interferes with my carrying out certain duties and responsibilities.	_____
8. Fatigue is among my three most disabling symptoms.	_____
9. Fatigue interferes with my work, family, or social life.	_____

Patients are instructed to choose a number from 1 to 7 that indicates their degree of agreement with each statement, in which 1 indicates strongly disagree, and 7, strongly agree.

(Reprinted with permission from Krupp LB, LaRocca NG, Muir-Nash J, Steinberg AD. The Fatigue Severity Scale: application to patients with multiple sclerosis and systemic lupus erythematosus. Arch Neurol 46:1121–1123, 1989.)

total of the responses, or be presented as the average score. The FSS has been shown to be effective for distinguishing fatigue in medically ill populations (systemic lupus erythematosus and MS) from those of healthy, nonfatigued controls.[2] In clinical trials of fatigue, it can detect positive treatment effects.[2,18–20]

While all self-report measures offer advantages in terms of ease of use, they also have obvious limitations in that all are subject to rater bias. They also require that the physician have the insight and ability to distinguish fatigue from other, often overlapping symptoms, such as depression and sleepiness. The scales all show varying degrees of fluctuation, with the VAS-F generally acknowledged as the most prone to variation. In addition, whereas longer scales, such as the FIS, MAF, or MFI, are multidimensional in nature, none of the available scales provides a truly accurate assessment of social, cognitive, or physical functioning, which can only be obtained by more extensive investigation into the patient's circumstances (e.g., by confirming work attendance through the patient's employer or assessing performance on neuropsychological tests).

There are a number of innovative methods of fatigue self-report that attempt to provide a more accurate assessment of fatigue. For example, ecological momentary assessment is a computerized, palm-top tool that assesses fatigue phenomena at various points throughout the day, and has been used to study fatigue in patients with CFS.[21] It has the advantage of using multiple repeated observations, which are typically made in the environments that patients inhabit. Patients are asked to respond to fatigue rating questionnaires using the palm-top device at several random moments throughout the day, as well as during certain events.

PERFORMANCE-BASED MEASUREMENTS

Performance-based measures, while less widely employed, can be useful under certain conditions and with certain diseases. They have the advantage of being more objective, as they are designed to measure abnormalities in muscle activation, central motor drive, and power output.[22] They are most often used in instances where fatigue may be localized to specific muscle groups (e.g., postpolio syndrome, MS, or amyotrophic lateral sclerosis).

Various measures of strength and endurance can be used in performance-based measurement. For example, in one study of 20 MS patients, myometry was used to test the isometric strength of seven muscle groups on both sides, including the elbow extensor, knee extensor, and ankle dorsiflexor. In addition, motor fatigue was assessed using three exercise protocols: sustained maximal contractions, repetitive maximal contractions, and a 500-meter walk.[23]

While performance-based measures have been shown to be reliable methods of assessing fatigue, they are more time-consuming and expensive. In addition, while they have greater objectivity than self-report scales, they are also subject to factors such as individual motivation or degree of effort.[22] Studies have also shown that they do not correlate well with subjective reports of fatigue.[24,25]

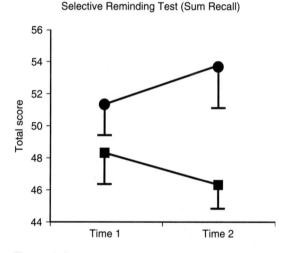

Figure 3-2. Verbal learning before (Time 1) and after (Time 2) a continuous cognitively effortful task in multiple sclerosis (MS) patients and controls. Circles indicate control subjects (n = 14); squares indicate patients with MS (n = 45). Group × Time: $F(1,57) = 2.96$, $p = 0.035$. (Reprinted with permission from Krupp LB, Elkins LE. Fatigue and declines in cognitive functioning in multiple sclerosis. Neurology 55:934–939, 2000.)

MEASUREMENT OF COGNITIVE FATIGUE

In addition to its effect on physical functioning, fatigue has also been associated with impairments in neuropsychologic and cognitive performance, engendering a great deal of interest in "cognitive fatigue" as a performance-based measure. One study showed that cognitive fatigue had a significant impact on verbal learning in MS patients, with patients undergoing a continuously effortful cognitive task (completing mental arithmetic problems on a computer) showing declines in measures of verbal memory and conceptual planning (Fig. 3-2).[26] Other studies have shown impairments in tests of memory, attention, and information processing in chronic fatigue syndrome patients irrespective of the presence of comorbid Axis I psychiatric disorders.[27]

CONCLUSIONS

Because there is significant overlap among fatigue and other illness features such as depression, pain, and excessive daytime sleepiness, it is good practice for physicians to employ other assessments in conjunction with fatigue measures. A version of the Visual Analog Scale for Pain (asking patients if they

Measurement of Fatigue: Key Concepts

- Fatigue can be measured either by self-reporting scales that assess the patient's perceived level of fatigue, or by performance-based measures that assess various neurophysiologic parameters such as muscle force generation.
- Various self-reporting scales are available, which can treat fatigue as either a single construct, or assess the impact of fatigue across multiple dimensions of functioning (e.g., physical and social).
- Self-reporting scales are advantageous in that they are easy to administer; however, they also have drawbacks in that they are subject to rater bias. They also require that the physician have the insight and ability to distinguish fatigue from other, often overlapping symptoms, such as depression and excessive daytime sleepiness.
- Performance-based measures of fatigue can be useful in instances in which fatigue is localized to specific muscle groups, which is often the case in certain disorders such as postpolio syndrome or multiple sclerosis. They can also be used in cases of "cognitive fatigue" to measure cognitive decrements over the course of performing tasks.
- Because of the overlap among fatigue and other illness features such as pain, depression, and excessive daytime sleepiness, the physician should also employ assessments of these symptoms in conjunction with fatigue measures.

feel pain on a scale of "no pain" to "pain as bad as can be") can be administered quickly and easily during each patient visit. The Epworth Sleepiness Scale, which assesses the patient's propensity to fall asleep under various nonstressful conditions (e.g., while reading or watching television) is a valuable tool for assessing excessive daytime sleepiness, and can be used to distinguish between symptoms of fatigue and sleepiness.[19] Finally, a number of common depression inventories, such as the Center for Epidemiologic Studies Depression Scale (CES-D),[28] the Hamilton Rating Scale for Depression (HAM-D),[29] and the Beck Depression Inventory[30] can be very helpful in assessing depressive symptoms.[31]

REFERENCES

1. Weinshenker BG, Penman M, Bass B, et al. A double-blind, randomized crossover trial of pemoline in fatigue associated with multiple sclerosis. Neurology 42:1468–1471, 1992.
2. Krupp LB, LaRocca NG, Muir-Nash J, Steinberg AD. The Fatigue Severity Scale: application to patients with multiple sclerosis and systemic lupus erythematosus. Arch Neurol 46:1121–1123, 1989.
3. Fisk JD, Ritvo PG, Ross L, et al. Measuring the impact of fatigue: initial validation of the Fatigue Impact Scale. Clin Infect Dis 18(suppl 1):S79–S83, 1994.

4. Multiple Sclerosis Clinical Practice Guideline: Fatigue and Multiple Sclerosis: Evidence-Based Management Strategies for Fatigue in Multiple Sclerosis. Washington, DC: Paralyzed Veterans Association, 1998.

5. Chalder T, Berelowitz G, Pawlikowska T, et al. Development of a fatigue scale. J Psychosom Res 37:147–153, 1993.

6. Belza BL, Henke CJ, Yelin EH, et al. Correlates of fatigue in older women with rheumatoid arthritis. Nurs Res 42:93–99, 1993.

7. Vercoulen J, Hommes OR, Swanink C, et al. The measurement of fatigue in patients with multiple sclerosis: a multidimensional comparison with patients with chronic fatigue syndrome and healthy subjects. Arch Neurol 53:642–649, 1996.

8. Smets EMA, Garssen B, Bonke B, De Haes JCJM. The Multidimensional Fatigue Inventory (MFI): psychometric qualities of an instrument to assess fatigue. J Psychosom Res 39:315–325, 1995.

9. Schwartz J, Jandorf L, Krupp LB. The measurement of fatigue: a new scale. J Psychosom Res 37:753–762, 1993.

10. Iriarte J, Katsamakis G, De Castro P. The fatigue descriptive scale (FDS): a useful tool to evaluate fatigue in multiple sclerosis. Mult Scler 5:10–16, 1999.

11. McNair DM, Lorr M, Droppleman LF. Profile of Mood States Manual (POMS). 2nd ed. San Diego, Calif: Educational and Industrial Testing Service, 1992.

12. Hann DM, Denniston MM, Baker F. Measurement of fatigue in cancer patients: further validation of

the Fatigue Symptom Inventory. Qual Life Res 9:847–854, 2000.

13. Ware JE, Kosinski M, Keller SD. SF-36 Physical and Mental Health Summary Scales: A User's Manual. Boston: The Health Institute, New England Medical Center, 1994.

14. Taylor RR, Jason LA, Torres A. Fatigue rating scales: an empirical comparison. Psychol Med 30:849–856, 2000.

15. LaChapelle DL, Finlayson MA. An evaluation of subjective and objective measures of fatigue in patients with brain injury and healthy controls. Brain Inj 12:649–659, 1998.

16. Belza BL. Comparison of self-reported fatigue in rheumatoid arthritis and controls. J Rheumatol 22:639–634, 1995.

17. Meek PM, Nail LM, Barsevick A, et al. Psychometric testing of fatigue instruments for use with cancer patients. Nurs Res 49:181–190, 2000.

18. Krupp LB, Coyle PK, Doscher C, et al. Fatigue therapy in multiple sclerosis: results of a double-blind, randomized, parallel trial of amantadine, pemoline, and placebo. Neurology 45:1956–1961, 1995.

19. Rammohan KW, Rosenberg JH, Lynn DJ, et al. Efficacy and safety of modafinil (Provigil) for the treatment of fatigue in multiple sclerosis: a two center phase 2 study. J Neurol Neurosurg Psychiatry 72:179–183, 2002.

20. Sheean G. Murray N, Rothwell J, et al. An open labeled clinical and electrophysiological study of 3,4 diaminopyridine in the treatment of fatigue in multiple sclerosis. Brain 121:967–975, 1998.

21. Stone AA, Broderick JE, Porter LS, et al. Fatigue and mood in chronic fatigue syndrome patients: results of a momentary assessment protocol examining fatigue and mood levels and diurnal patterns. Ann Behav Med 16:228–234, 1994.

22. Elkins LE, Krupp LB, Scherl W. The measurement of fatigue and contributing neuropsychiatric factors. Semin Clin Neuropsychiatry 5:58–61, 2000.

23. Schwid SR, Thornton CA, Pandya S, et al. Quantitative assessment of motor fatigue and strength in MS. Neurology 53:743–750, 1999.

24. Marshall PS, Watson D, Steinberg P, et al. An assessment of cognitive function and mood in chronic fatigue syndrome. Biol Psych 39:199–206, 1996.

25. Stein DP, Dambrosia JM, Dalakas MC. A double-blind, placebo-controlled trial of amantadine for the treatment of fatigue in patients with the post-polio syndrome. Ann N Y Acad Sci 753:296–302, 1995.

26. Krupp LB, Elkins LE. Fatigue and declines in cognitive functioning in multiple sclerosis. Neurology 55:934–939, 2000.

27. DeLuca J, Johnson SK, Ellis SP, Natelson BH. Cognitive functioning is impaired in patients with chronic fatigue syndrome devoid of psychiatric illness. J Neurol Neurosurg Psychiatry 62:151–155, 1997.

28. Radloff LS. CES-D scale: A self-report depression scale for research in the general population. Appl Psychol Meas 1:385–401, 1977.

29. Patten CA, Gillin JC, Golshan S, et al. Relationship of mood disturbance to cigarette smoking status

among 252 patients with a current mood disorder. J Clin Psychiatry 62:319-324, 2001 May.

30. Beck AT, Ward CH, Mendelson M. An inventory for measuring depression. Arch Gen Psych 4:561–571, 1961.

31. Cassano GB, Puca F, Scapicchio PL, Trabucchi M. Paroxetine and fluoxetine effects on mood and cognitive functions in depressed nondemented elderly patients. J Clin Psychiatry 63:396–402, 2002.

CHAPTER FOUR

Fatigue Covariables

Fatigue is rarely an isolated symptom of any disease. Usually, it appears in conjunction with other symptoms. Common covariates of fatigue include sleep disorders, pain, mood disturbance, and symptoms of cognitive difficulty. In some cases, the symptom of fatigue is misleading, mimicking a different primary problem. For example, in a sleep disorder such as narcolepsy, diagnosing and treating the sleep problem is all that is necessary to treat the fatigue. More often, the symptoms of mood disturbance, sleepiness, pain, and fatigue overlap and exacerbate one another. Because these covariates may also impede treatment efforts designed to reduce fatigue, it is important for the physician to have a high index of suspicion for the many related problems that are experienced by the fatigued patient.

SLEEP DISORDERS

Daytime fatigue often coexists with sleep disorders.[1] For example, it has been observed that two thirds of systemic lupus erythematosus (SLE) patients report poor sleep quality, and that sleep problems correlate with fatigue in these patients.[2] Excessive daytime sleepiness is also common in patients with movement disorders such as Parkinson's disease. In these patients, motor manifestations of disease, such as periodic limb movements of sleep, interfere with sleep activity, causing daytime fatigue. Interruption in sleep patterns leading to daytime fatigue can also be caused by conditions such as sleep apnea syndrome.

In the author's experience, on rare occasions a patient presenting with severe fatigue will, on closer inspection, give a history of very disrupted sleep or sudden episodes of abruptly falling asleep.[3] In these cases, polysomnography can lead to a primary sleep diagnosis and appropriate intervention will resolve the fatigue. In other cases of patients with severe fatigue and abnormalities on polysomnography, a distinct diagnosis of a particular sleep disorder may be less straightforward.

It is important to try to determine the basis for reports of sleepiness in the fatigued patient. Often, the patient's bed partner is the most valuable resource for diagnosing a sleep disorder. The history should include querying the bed partner about the presence of disrupted sleep patterns or apneas/hypopneas. The Epworth Sleepiness Scale is an excellent tool to assess the degree of excessive daytime sleepiness (Table 4-1); a score of ≥ 10 indicates the presence of excessive daytime sleepiness. Referral to

Table 4-1. Epworth Sleepiness Scale

Indicate your chance of falling asleep under the following situations:
0 = no chance of dozing
1 = slight chance of dozing
2 = moderate chance of dozing
3 = high chance of dozing

Situation	*Chance of Dozing*
Sitting and reading	_____
Watching TV	_____
Sitting inactive in a public place (e.g., a theater or a meeting)	_____
As a passenger in a car for an hour without a break	_____
Lying down to rest in the afternoon when circumstances permit	_____
Sitting and talking to someone	_____
Sitting quietly after a lunch without alcohol	_____
In a car, while stopped for a few minutes in traffic	_____

a sleep clinic may be appropriate for certain sleep disorders such as obstructive sleep apnea or narcolepsy. Patients who continue to experience excessive daytime sleepiness or fatigue despite treatment of an underlying sleep disorder may benefit from use of a wake-promoting agent such as modafinil.

PAIN

Pain and fatigue have a high degree of overlap, and it is often difficult for patients to determine which of these two symptoms has the greatest effect on functioning.[4] There are numerous reasons why pain contributes to fatigue. Physically, pain can cause deconditioning by limiting activity. The presence of nighttime pain can cause excessive daytime sleepiness and fatigue by interfering with the patient's normal sleep patterns. Pain also has a high degree of association with psychological factors. It can contribute to depression or other affective disorders, and these can, in turn, increase feelings of fatigue. Finally, it is likely that the experience of moving and functioning in pain is energy consuming and leads to a depletion of reserves.

Pain commonly occurs with fatigue in movement disorders such as Parkinson's disease, as well as other disorders that cause severe physical limitations such as postpolio syndrome, multiple sclerosis (MS), or arthritic conditions such as rheumatoid arthritis or SLE. In these patients, pain resulting from joint swelling, or the constant strain of unwanted muscle activity such as tremor and spasticity, can be difficult to overcome. However, pain is also a typical symptom in "unexplained clinical conditions" such as fibromyalgia, chronic fatigue syndrome (CFS), and irritable bowel syndrome.[5] In these patients, it is important to keep in mind that pain can occur independent of physical factors. For example, in fibromyalgia patients, it has been shown that pain can be brought on by mental strain—a type of "painful exhaustion."[4,6]

Like fatigue, pain can be assessed by self-report measures such as a visual analog scale. Pain resulting from a definite physical cause (e.g., constant muscle rigidity) can be treated with appropriate analgesics and muscle relaxants. Pain without an identifiable physical cause is more of a treatment challenge, and it may be helpful to address other potential underlying causes, such as depression.

DEPRESSION/PSYCHOSOCIAL STATE

Affective disorders such as depression are very common among fatigue patients. Fatigue is a typical symptom of depression, and is often reported as a lack of motivation or energy. Depression can be brought on by fatigue, and it can in turn engender additional fatigue (Fig. 4-1).[7]

An association between fatigue and depression has been reported in a number of disorders, including CFS and MS.[8] It is also common in Parkinson's disease and has been shown to correlate strongly with fatigue in people with epilepsy.[9] Fatigue is a major component of a number of affective disorders, including major depression, seasonal affective disorder, and dysthymia.[1]

There are numerous theories as to why depression is common in persons with fatigue. In disorders such as MS, in which there is a clear insult to

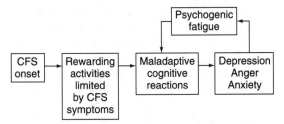

Figure 4-1. Model of affective distress in CFS. (Reprinted with permission from Friedberg F, Krupp LB. A comparison of cognitive behavioral treatment for chronic fatigue syndrome and primary depression. Clin Infect Dis 18[suppl 1]:S105–S110, 1994.)

the neurologic system, depression and fatigue may stem from damage to the same neurologic pathways. In addition, it is possible that the depression itself can be the main cause of the patient's symptoms. In support of this, growing evidence exists that depression can lead to functional disability and somatization.[10] In CFS especially, there has been a high degree of speculation that most cases of disease are in fact cases of depression or somatization disorder.[7] This is likely to be true in some patients but does not apply to all patients. It is just as likely that depression will be a consequence, and not the antecedent, of chronic fatigue.

Depression can also be the result of the stresses associated with chronic illness, as has been reported in SLE.[2] These stresses can increase depression, to the point that depression can replace the underlying disease as the patient's primary concern. Finally, depression in chronic fatigue has been linked to changes in neurohormonal or immunologic function. A growing body of research supports a relationship between stressful life events and psychologic distress, and impairments in cellular immunity.[10]

Regardless of the cause, depression in the fatigue patient must be addressed. Treatment for depression may be helpful for reducing fatigue symptoms in CFS as well as other disorders. Cognitive behavioral therapy is the most effective therapy to date shown to help both fatigue and depression symptoms in chronic fatigue patients.[7,11] Often the addition of an antidepressant can be helpful.

Psychosocial factors can also contribute significantly to the patient's perceived fatigue severity.[12] For example, in SLE patients fatigue has been associated with higher levels of perceived helplessness, as well as the lack of health insurance.[12] Similarly in MS, feelings of control lessen fatigue, whereas focusing on bodily sensations can exacerbate fatigue.[13] Individuals who feel they can create environments appropriate to their psychologic and physical needs experience less fatigue and fatigue-related stress.[14] In other medical groups who experience severe fatigue, fatigue correlates with low positive affect but does not correspond with elevated negative affect.[15,16]

COGNITIVE DEFICITS

Reports of cognitive difficulties are common in patients with symptoms of fatigue. However symptoms of cognitive dysfunction do not always indicate cognitive impairment.[14,17] For example, improvement in mood reduces complaints of poor memory in individuals who are depressed,[17] whereas in patients with MS, reports of marked cognitive difficulty are more likely to be associated with relatively intact performance on cognitive tests but elevated scores on depression inventories. In contrast, MS patients with moderate levels of reported problems show more congruent test performance consistent with moderate impairments.[8]

The association between perceived cognitive problems and mood disturbance has also been observed in human immunodeficiency virus (HIV) infection. Memory complaints in HIV-infected adults can be attributed both to impairments in frontal lobe executive function, as well as mood disturbance.[18] These studies clearly demonstrate that the fatigued patient often has symptoms of memory problems or verbal fluency, and that these complaints require further assessment to interpret their meaning. The additional evaluation should include assessment of both mood as well as formal cognitive test performance. Relying on symptoms alone can be misleading.

Relatively little is known about whether the mechanisms responsible for fatigue overlap with brain disturbances that can lead to cognitive dysfunction. As with depression, however, it is possible that cognitive deficits and fatigue may arise from insults along common neurologic pathways. Coexistent depression may also lead to difficulties

Fatigue Covariables: Key Concepts

- Fatigue is rarely an isolated symptom of any disease; instead, it commonly appears in conjunction with symptoms such as sleep disorders, pain, mood disorders, or cognitive dysfunction.
- Daytime fatigue is often a coexistent feature of sleep disorders, such as restless legs syndrome, sleep apnea syndrome, or narcolepsy. Sleep testing in the form of a self-report scale or referral to a sleep clinic may be helpful in identifying sleep disorders.
- Pain and fatigue have a high degree of overlap, and pain can contribute to fatigue by limiting activity, interfering with sleep, or causing depression. The physician should specifically ask about the presence of pain and take steps to relieve pain in the fatigued patient.
- Fatigue is often a symptom of an affective disorder such as depression. Depression can be the main cause of the patient's fatigue symptoms, or the result of stresses associated with chronic illness. It may also be the result of damage to the same neurologic pathways that cause fatigue.
- Reports of cognitive difficulties are common in patients with fatigue. Symptoms of cognitive difficulty may be the result of a coexistent mood disorder. To distinguish cognitive complaints from deficits in executive functioning, formal cognitive testing may be needed. If a mood disorder such as depression is present, treating the mood disorder may help improve cognitive symptoms.

in cognitive processing, mentation, and attention span. Awareness of the association between cognitive problems and fatigue is important because of the need to rely on self-report scales in fatigue diagnosis. Patients who show significant difficulty with cognition may benefit from being given more time to fill out fatigue assessment scales or a more detailed explanation of how to complete the scales.

CONCLUSIONS

Symptoms of fatigue do not occur in a vacuum, and the treating physician should be aware of the associations among fatigue, cognitive complaints (versus cognitive deficits), depression, pain, and sleep disorders. All of these factors may contribute to the patient's total burden of illness, and treatment of one symptom may reduce the symptom severity of other symptoms.

REFERENCES

1. Morrison RE, Keating HJ. Fatigue in primary care. Obstet Gynecol Clin North Am 28:225–237, 2001.
2. Tench CM, McCurdie I, White PD, Cruz DP. The prevalence and associations of fatigue in systemic lupus erythematosus. Rheumatology 39:1249–1254, 2000.

3. Krupp LB, Mendelson WB, Friedman R. An overview of chronic fatigue syndrome. J Clin Psychiatry 52:403–410, 1991.

4. Wessely S, Hotopf M, Sharpe M. Chronic Fatigue and its Syndromes. London: Oxford University Press, 1999.

5. Aaron LA, Buchwald D. A review of the evidence for overlap among unexplained clinical conditions. Ann Intern Med 134:868–881, 2001.

6. Bansevicius D, Westgaard RH, Stiles T. EMG activity and pain development in fibromyalgia patients exposed to mental stress of long duration. Scand J Rheumatol 30:92–98, 2001.

7. Friedberg F, Krupp LB. A comparison of cognitive behavioral treatment for chronic fatigue syndrome and primary depression. Clin Infect Dis 18(suppl 1):S105–S110, 1994.

8. Schwartz CE, Coulthard-Morris L, Zeng Q. Psychosocial correlates of fatigue in multiple sclerosis. Arch Phys Med Rehabil 77:165–170, 1996.

9. Ettinger AB, Weisbrot DM, Krupp LB, et al. Fatigue and depression in epilepsy. J Epilepsy 11:105–109, 1998.

10. Katon WY, Buchwald DS, Simon GE, Russo JE, Mease PJ. Psychiatric illness in patients with chronic fatigue and those with rheumatoid arthritis. J Gen Intern Med 6:277–285, 1991.

11. Whiting P, Bagnall AM, Sowden AJ, et al. Interventions for the treatment and management of chronic fatigue syndrome: a systematic review. JAMA 286:1360–1368, 2001.

12. Zonana-Nacach A, Roseman JM, McGwin G, et al. Systemic lupus erythematosus in three ethnic

groups, VI: factors associated with fatigue within 5 years of criteria diagnosis. Lupus 9:101, 2000.

13. Vercoulen J, Hommes OR, Swanink C, et al. The measurement of fatigue in patients with multiple sclerosis: a multidimensional comparison with patients with chronic fatigue syndrome and healthy subjects. Arch Neurol 53:642–649, 1996.

14. Schwartz CE, Kozora E, Zeng Q. Towards patient collaboration in cognitive assessment: specificity, sensitivity, and incremental validity of self-report. Ann Behav Med 18:177–184, 1996.

15. Elkins LE, Pollina DA, Scheffer S, Krupp LB. Psychological states and neuropsychological performances in chronic Lyme disease. Appl Neuropsych 6:19–26, 1999.

16. Marshall PS, Watson D, Steinberg P, et al. An assessment of cognitive function and mood in chronic fatigue syndrome. Biol Psych 39:199–206, 1996.

17. Antikainen R, Hanninen T, Honkalampi K, et al. Mood improvement reduces memory complaints in depressed patients. Eur Arch Psych Clin Neurosci 251:6–11, 2001.

18. Rourke SB, Halman MH, Bassel C. Neuropsychiatric correlates of memory-metamemory dissociations in HIV infection. J Clin Exp Neuropsych 21:757–768, 1999.

Fatigue Pathophysiology

Because of the complexity of fatigue and its occurrence in such a wide variety of disorders, it is unlikely that any one pathophysiologic cause can explain fatigue in all patients. Nonetheless, some common pathophysiologic mechanisms of fatigue have been explored across several diseases. Likely factors related to fatigue include dysfunction across neuroanatomic pathways, alterations in the feedback processes related to the endocrine system, abnormalities in the immune responses, and a combination of chronic illness and psychological factors.

In some diseases fatigue has been linked to energy depletion. For example, in postoperative states and in cancer, factors responsible for fatigue include excessive metabolic demands, anemia, and cachexia, all direct consequence of the underlying condition. Some of these disease-specific fatigue mechanisms are covered in more detail under the specific disorders (e.g., cancer) but the common mechanisms reviewed in this chapter overlap with those specific to particular disorders and are not mutually exclusive. In fact, most likely there is substantial interplay among different mechanisms for fatigue in any given patient. This chapter provides a brief overview of several concepts regarding fatigue pathophysiology for which there is some empiric support.

CENTRAL NERVOUS SYSTEM MECHANISMS

A number of distinct central nervous system (CNS) disorders include fatigue as a major symptom. Among the CNS regions in which dysfunction is believed to contribute to fatigue development are the premotor cortex, the limbic system, the basal ganglia, and the brain-stem areas. Dysfunction in these areas could lead to decreased motivation or motor readiness, which could relate to fatigue. However, there are no studies to suggest a single lesion or neuroanatomic structural abnormality within the brain is solely responsible for fatigue.[1,2]

In the CNS disorder multiple sclerosis (MS), fatigue is considered to be a consequence of dysfunction either related to the demyelination of nerve sheaths and destruction of axons within the brain or spinal cord, or a result of immune changes affecting the brain and spinal cord. Fatigue also is prevalent in Parkinson's disease, another CNS disorder in which patients experience significant, progressive neurologic damage. In both of these disorders, fatigue has been associated with reduced frontal lobe activity, characterized by deficits in perfusion and glucose uptake.[3,4] Fatigue may also be associated with a failure of motor functions within the basal ganglia and pathways involving the striatal-thalamic-frontal cortical system.[5]

On the other hand, the hypothalamus and pathways involving neurotransmitters such as dopamine, histamine, and serotonin, are also likely to contribute to fatigue pathogenesis. For example, it has been argued that disruption in serotonergic pathways interferes with attention, and could lead to cognitive fatigue.[6,7] Effects on the hypothalamus can lead to decreased arousal and hence increased fatigue.

It may be that fatigue as a symptom depends on defects in both neuroendocrine and neurotransmitter systems, as well as the interactions between these systems. There are sufficient data to demonstrate that disruption of the neuroendocrine axis may be related to perceived stress, arousal, and fatigue.[8] Furthermore, given that studies have correlated altered cerebral metabolism with fatigue,[3] it is reasonable to conclude that a decrease in the brain supply of glucose via decreased blood glucose or impaired cerebral glucose metabolism could underlie fatigue.

NEUROMUSCULAR FACTORS

Peripheral fatigue, or fatigue defined as any reduction of maximal muscle force or motor output, has been associated with disorders of motor control including impaired muscular excitation, contraction, and metabolism.[9,10] However, in most studies to date, the objective documentation of motor fatiguability does not correspond to perceived or subjective fatigue. For example, the muscle fatigue experienced by amytrophic lateral sclerosis (ALS) patients is not correlated with subjective feelings of fatigue[9]; and measures of intracellular metabolism and muscle physiology during maximum voluntary contraction of the tibialis anterior muscle are also not significantly different in patients with severe fatigue and unfatigued healthy controls.[11] At present, the way abnormalities in motor pathways are associated with fatigue are unclear and do not appear directly causally responsible for the subjective experience of fatigue.[12]

ENDOCRINE SYSTEM DYSFUNCTION

A significant degree of research has been focused on the endocrine system in the development of fatigue, especially the role of the hypothalamic-pituitary-adrenal (HPA) axis, which is the body's stress regulator. In response to stress, the hypothalamus releases corticotrophin-releasing factor (CRF), which triggers the release of adrenocorticotrophic hormone (ACTH) from the pituitary gland. ACTH acts on the adrenal cortex, causing it to release cortisol in the bloodstream. Cortisol exerts a negative feedback effect on the hypothalamus to inhibit further CRF release and thus reduce cortisol levels.

Support for a significant role of the HPA axis in fatigue pathophysiology is found in the fact that the course of chronic fatigue syndrome (CFS) often is exacerbated by physical and emotional stressors.[13] Studies have shown diminished activity in the HPA axis in persons with CFS and idiopathic pain syndromes such as fibromyalgia and irritable bowel syndrome. These data show a reduced activation of the adrenal gland, with low circulating levels of cortisol, which is highly sensitive to stress.[14]

Although HPA axis dysregulation appears to play some causative role in the development of fatigue, there are a number of issues that require further exploration. It is not clear whether endocrine dysfunction is a primary cause of fatigue, or whether the reduction in cortisol levels occurs secondary to some other cause such as changes in sleep or exercise. (Exercise can upregulate cortisol levels, and the deconditioning that occurs from lack of exercise in fatigue patients may make cortisol levels chronically low.)

Also, although cortisol reductions in chronic fatigue are present, the degree of reduction is generally far from remarkable, and there is not an impressive correlation between cortisol levels and fatigue severity or chronicity.[15] For example, many patients with CFS continue to have cortisol levels which, although low, still fall well within normal ranges. As a whole, the evidence does not support dysregulation of any single endocrine pathway as the major pathophysiologic mechanism that drives chronic fatigue symptomatology. In recognition of this, cortisol levels are not used as a diagnostic marker for CFS.[16]

Additional endocrine pathways related to fatigue include the regulation of growth hormone, thyroid function, and gonadal axis hypoactivity. Studies in different populations have demonstrated the association between fatigue and gonadal function. For example, in a study of hormonal ablative treatment in cancer of the prostate, a direct link between fatigue and gonadrotropin function was observed.[17] Furthermore, in some cases treatments designed to increase hormone levels such as testosterone may result in decreased fatigue.[18,19] Decreased gonadotropin levels are also associated with poor appetite and cachexia. Hence the fatigue associated with gonadotropin changes could be indirect and result from other physiologic changes related to gonadotropin function that could worsen fatigue.

IMMUNOLOGIC FACTORS

There are several lines of evidence that suggest immune system dysregulation plays a role in fatigue. First, medications that are products of the immune system, such as cytokines, when given to patients with different disorders, clearly produce fatigue as a side effect. For example, high-dose interleukin-2 administration causes fatigue, fever, and myalgia.[20] In addition, both interferon α and interferon β can induce fatigue, as well as other neuropsychiatric complications.[21,22]

Second, fatigue is a prominent symptom in disorders of autoimmune cause such as systemic lupus erythemoatosus and MS. In both disorders, patients may experience episodes of severe fatigue as part of a disease exacerbation or relapse, and fatigue can develop prior to signs of organ damage.

Finally, a range of different perturbations in the immune response has been identified in individuals with persistent and severe fatigue. For example, in fatigued patients with CFS, several changes consistent with a decreased cellular immunity have been identified.[15] Increases in the number of activated T lymphocytes has been reported, as well as increased numbers of cytokines such as interleukin 1 and tumor necrosis factor (TNF)-α, which have effects on sleep regulation and are involved in sleep-related disorders such as sleep apnea and idiopathic hypersomnia. Evidence also suggests that these cytokines accumulate during periods of wakefulness and promote fatigue.[15]

Elevations in TNF-α have also been linked to fatigue in patients undergoing dialylsis.[23] Even in healthy adults, cytokines can produce fatigue. In a study of 16 healthy males, administration of the cytokine IL-6 produced increased fatigue and changes in sleep architecture.[24] Because IL-6 had its effects independently of changes in interferon α and interferon γ, it appears that even though cytokines induce one another they can have independent effects on fatigue.

An association between perceived fatigue and circulating markers of immune activation has also been observed in MS patients.[25] Others examining inflammatory cytokines and fatigue have not replicated these findings.[26] Given the sensitivity of circulating inflammatory cytokines to so many variables, and the difficulties and multiple factors affecting measurement of cytokine levels, it is not surprising that linking cytokines or other biologic markers of immune activation with such a heterogeneous entity as fatigue would be difficult.

Despite the possible contribution of activation of the immune system and fatigue, it appears that immune cell function in chronically fatigued patients is poor, with low natural killer cell cytotoxicity, a poor lymphocyte response, and frequent immunoglobulin deficiencies.[27] However, these immune changes are not specific enough for diagnostic purposes and are not correlated with end organ damage in chronically fatigued individuals.[16]

It has been suggested that immune system activation exerts an effect on the neuroendocrine system, with cytokines promoting the secretion of CRF, ACTH, and cortisol.[15] Interferons may mediate fatigue through effects on thyroid function. Autoimmune thyroid disease is a known consequence of interferon therapy. In addition, interferon administration can alter antigen expression in the thyroid and lead to thyroiditis.[28] The reverse may also be true, with HPA axis dysregulation having an effect on immune cell activation and the inflammatory process. Thus, it is unclear whether neuroendocrine dysfunction may represent the "final common pathway" for fatigue.

AUTONOMIC NERVOUS SYSTEM DYSFUNCTION

There is growing evidence that reduced autonomic nervous system activity contributes at least in part to fatigue.[29] Recent studies have suggested a connection between autonomic regulation of blood pressure and chronic fatigue. Many CFS patients experience lightheadedness and a worsening of fatigue when standing for prolonged periods, symptoms that are also characteristic of neurally mediated hypotension. From the standpoint of intervention, treatment of neurally mediated hypotension has been associated with improvements in fatigue in CFS patients (although not all studies show an improvement in chronic fatigue symptoms with the use of the mineralocorticoid fludrocortisone).[30,31]

It is likely that hypofunctionality of the autonomic nervous system, even when present, is not the primary cause of fatigue symptoms. For example, reduced HPA-axis activity has been associated with an overall impairment in central nervous system drive.[13] Questions remain regarding the extent to which autonomic system dysfunction impacts other disorders in which fatigue is a symptom. For example, a recent study showed moderate to severe cardiovascular autonomic abnormalities in more than one quarter of MS patients.[32] However, the overall contribution to fatigue was considered minimal.

THE INFLUENCE OF PSYCHOLOGICAL FACTORS

There is a complex relationship between fatigue and various psychological factors, making it difficult to determine the extent to which psychological symptoms such as depression and anxiety either cause or contribute to fatigue. Clearly, fatigue is a hallmark symptom of depression and anxiety disorders, and stress, anxiety, and poor coping strategies in response to difficult situations can all contribute to fatigue. Importantly, fatigue is a common complaint in those with somatization disorder (the experience of physical symptoms as a result of psychological distress). Studies have shown that as many as one third of hospitalized chronic fatigue patients fulfill criteria for somatization disorder,[33] although the prevalence is lower in primary care populations.[15]

Psychological vulnerability may also predispose the individual to prolonged recoveries from viral infection or other illnesses and may exacerbate fatigue or lead to its persistence. Early work suggesting a relationship between persistent fatigue and psychological vulnerability was conducted in prospective studies of military personnel at risk for developing Asian Flu. In the late 1950s, investigators noted that elevated scores of depression and loss of morale as shown on the Minnesota Multiphasic Personality Inventory (MMPI) were associated with delayed recovery from the flu.[34,35] Elevated MMPI scores were associated with a higher incidence of hypersensitivity reactions to prophylactic inoculation.[36] A landmark study in the 1990s showed that levels of perceived stress in healthy volunteers before inoculation with live viruses were associated with an increased susceptibility in clinical syndromes of upper respiratory infection.[37] Of 394 volunteers exposed to one of several viruses that produce upper respiratory infection, those with higher levels of perceived stress before the inoculation were more likely to develop clinical evidence of a cold as stress levels increased. Similarly, the proportion of subjects with colds was notably less at the lower stress levels (fewer than 30% had colds) compared with the highest levels (in which approximately 45% had colds). These findings suggest that psychological factors and stress may predispose to the development of illness and may support the concept that such factors could produce persistent fatigue after a viral infection.

Consistent with this notion is the observation that postviral fatigue can be associated with increased psychological stress and attributional style.[38] Thus, psychological vulnerability, attributional style, and coping are important mechanisms in persistent fatigue and apply to medical disorders.

Psychological stress may potentially act by interfering with HPA-axis activity, or it may have an effect on immunologic responses. Although the connection between stress and persistent fatigue is not conclusive, psychological stress has been shown to increase markers of immunologic activity (e.g., in women experiencing marital disruption).[39] The risk of developing fatigue also appears to be much higher in persons who work in "difficult" psychosocial environments compared with those who work in more favorable environments.[15]

CONCLUSIONS

The pathophysiologic mechanisms behind fatigue are poorly understood and vary across different

Fatigue Pathophysiology: Key Concepts

- Although the pathophysiology of fatigue is not fully understood, mechanisms have been identified that may be common to fatigue in a number of disease states.
- Fatigue has been linked to energy depletion in some diseases, such as postoperative fatigue and cancer. Fatigue in these cases may be related to excessive metabolic demands placed on the body as a result of the body's efforts to cope with the injury or disease.
- Fatigue has been linked to central nervous system dysfunction in several disorders, including multiple sclerosis (MS) and Parkinson's disease. In these cases, fatigue may be related to deficits in nerve conduction, reduced frontal lobe activity and basal ganglia function, and disruption in neurotransmitter (i.e., serotonergic) or neuroendocrine pathways.
- Fatigue may be related to endocrine system dysfunction, especially dysregulation of the hypothalamic-pituitary-adrenal (HPA) axis, which is the body's stress regulator. Chronically low levels of cortisol resulting from HPA-axis dysregulation may be a primary cause of fatigue, or related to some secondary factor such as changes in sleep or exercise habits.
- Immune system dysregulation may play a role in fatigue, either directly or through mediation of neuroendocrine function. Nevertheless, studies of immune markers (e.g., interleukin 1, tumor

(continued)

Fatigue Pathophysiology: Key Concepts—Cont'd

---

necrosis factor α) have failed to identify a single immunologic factor or group of factors that can consistently explain fatigue.

- There is growing evidence that autonomic nervous system dysfunction may play a role in fatigue development. Studies have shown a connection between autonomic regulation of blood pressure and chronic fatigue.

- Psychological factors such as depression and anxiety may be at least partially responsible for the emergence of fatigue symptoms. In addition, a state of psychological vulnerability or chronic stress (e.g., in persons experiencing abuse or marital difficulties) may exacerbate fatigue or lead to its persistence.

---

diseases, although some common underlying mechanisms do exist. Fatigue most likely represents a physiologic adaptation of the organism to a weakened internal condition unable to meet external demands. It is also likely that a complex interaction of neurotransmitters, neurohormones, immune factors, products of energy utilization (e.g., ATP), chronic illness factors, and psychological factors contribute to the fatigue experience. The exploration of animal models for fatigue also provides another opportunity for future research to address this overwhelming yet still poorly understood problem. Better defined research studies that consider different models of fatigue, address various fatigue subtypes, examine common features of fatigue across diverse medical conditions, and employ a range of measurement approaches will help provide better paradigms for understanding this complex multivariated phenomenon.

REFERENCES

1. Bakshi R, Miletich RS, Hanschel K, et al. Fatigue in multiple sclerosis: cross-sectional correlation with brain MRI findings in 71 patients. Neurology 53:1151–1153, 1999.
2. Mainero C, Faroni J, Gasperini C, et al. Fatigue and magnetic resonance imaging activity in multiple sclerosis. J Neurol 246:454–458, 1999.
3. Roelcke U, Kappos L, Lechner-Scott J, et al. Reduced glucose metabolism in the frontal cortex and basal ganglia of multiple sclerosis patients with fatigue: a 18F-fluorodeoxyglucose positron emission tomography study. Neurology 48: 1566–1571, 1997.
4. Abe K, Takanashi M, Yanagihara T. Fatigue in patients with Parkinson's disease. Behav Neurol 12:103–106, 2000.
5. Chadhuri A, Behan PO. Fatigue and basal ganglia. J Neurol Sci 179(suppl 1–2):34–42, 2000.
6. Parker AJ, Wessely S, Cleare AJ. The neuroendocrinology of chronic fatigue syndrome

and fibromyalgia. Psychol Med 31: 1331–1345, 2001.

7. Heilman KM, Watson RT. Fatigue. Neurology Network Commentary 1:283–287, 1997.

8. Wei T, Lightman SL. The neuroendocrine axis in patients with multiple sclerosis. Brain 120: 1067–1076, 1997.

9. Sharma KR, Kent-Braun JA, Majumdar S, et al. Physiology of fatigue in amyotrophic lateral sclerosis. Neurology 45:733–740, 1995.

10. Sharma KR, Mynhier MA, Miller RG. Muscular fatigue in Duchenne muscular dystrophy. Neurology 45:306–310, 1995.

11. Kent-Braun JA, Sharma KR, Weiner MW, et al. Central basis of muscle fatigue in chronic fatigue syndrome. Neurology 43:125–131, 1993.

12. Rutherford OM, White PD. Human quadriceps strength and fatiguability in patients with post viral fatigue. J Neurol Neurosurg Psychiatry 54:961–964, 1991.

13. Demitrack MA, Crofford LJ. Evidence for and pathophysiologic implications of hypothalamic-pituitary-adrenal axis dysregulation in fibromyalgia and chronic fatigue syndrome. Ann NY Acad Sci 840:684–697, 1998.

14. Ehlert U, Gaab J, Henrichs M. Psychoneuroen-docrinological contributions to the etiology of depression, posttraumatic stress disorder, and stress-related bodily disorders: the role of the hypothalamus-pituitary-adrenal axis. Biol Psychiatry 57:141–152, 2001.

15. Wessely S, Hotopf M, Sharpe M. Chronic Fatigue and its Syndromes. London: Oxford University Press, 1999.

16. Centers for Disease Control. Possible causes of CFS. Available at: http://www.cdc.gov/ncidod/diseases/cfs/causes.htm. Last accessed: July 10, 2002.

17. Stone P. Fatigue in patients with prostate cancer receiving hormone therapy. Eur J Cancer 36:1134–1141, 2000.

18. Rabkin JG, Ferrando SJ, Wagner GJ, Rabkin R. DHEA treatment of HIV+ patients: effects on mood, androgenic and anabolic parameters. Psychoneuroendocrinology 25: 53–68, 2000.

19. Wagner GJ, Rabkin JG, Rabkin R. Testosterone as a treatment for HIV+ men. Gen Hosp Psychiatry 20:209–213, 1998.

20. Denicoff KD, Durkin TM, Lotze MT, et al. The neuroendocrine effects of interleukin-2 treatment. J Clin Endocrinol Metab 69:402–410, 1989.

21. Quesada JR, Talpax M, Rios A, et al. Clinical toxicity of interferons in cancer patients: a review. J Clin Oncol 4:234–243, 1986.

22. Neilly LK, Goodin DS, Goodkin DE, Hause SL. Side effect profile of interferon beta-1b in MS: results of an open label trial. Neurology 46:552–554, 1996.

23. Dreisback AW, Hendrickson T, Beezhold D, et al. Elevated levels of tumor necrosis factor alpha in postdialysis fatigue. Int J Artific Organs 21: 83–86, 1998.

24. Spath-Schwalbe E, Hansen K, Schmidt F, et al. Acute effects of recombinant human interleukin-6 on encodcrine and central nervous sleep functions in healthy men. J Clin Endocrinol Metab 83:1573–1579, 1998.

25. Iriarte J, Subira ML, Castro P. Modalities of fatigue in multiple sclerosis: correlation with clinical and biological factors. Mult Scler 6:124–130, 2000.

26. Giovannoni G, Thompson AJ, Miller DH, Thompson EJ. Fatigue is not associated with raised inflammatory markers in multiple sclerosis. Neurology 57:676–681, 2001.

27. Patarca R. Cytokines and chronic fatigue syndrome. Ann NY Acad Sci 933:185–200, 2001.

28. Jones TH, Wadler S, Hupart KH. Endocrine mediated mechanisms of fatigue during treatment with interferon-alpha. Semin Oncol 25(supp I): 54–63, 1998.

29. Neeck G, Crofford LJ. Neuroendocrine perturbations in fibromyalgia and chronic fatigue syndrome. Rheum Dis Clin North Am 26:989–1002, 2000.

30. Rowe PC, Calkins H, DeBusk K, et al. Fludrocortisone acetate to treat neurally mediated hypotension in chronic fatigue syndrome: a randomized controlled trial. JAMA 285:52–59, 2001.

31. Rowe PC, Calkins H. Neurally mediated hypotension and chronic fatigue syndrome. Am J Med 105(suppl 3A):15S–21S, 1998.

32. Merkelbach S, Dillman U, Kolmel C, et al. Cardiovascular autonomic dysregulation and fatigue in multiple sclerosis. Mult Scler 7:320–326, 2001.

33. Farmer A, Jones I, Hillier J, et al. Neuraesthenia revisited: *ICD-10* and *DSM-III-R* psychiatric syndromes in chronic fatigue patients and comparison subjects. Br J Psychiatry 167: 503–506, 1995.

34. Imboden JB, Canter A, Cluff LE, Trevor RW. Brucellosis: psychological aspects of delayed convalescence. Arch Intern Med 103: 404–444, 1959.

35. Imboden JB, Canter A, Cluff LE. Convalescence from influenza: a study of the psychological and clinical determinants. Arch Intern Med 108:393–399, 1961.

36. Canter A, Cluff LE, Imboden JB. Hypersensitive reactions to immunization inoculations and antecedent psychological vulnerability. J Psychosom Res 16:99–101, 1972.

37. Cohen S, Tyrrell AJ, Smith AP. Psychological stress and susceptibility to the common cold. N Engl J Med 325:606–612, 1991.

38. Cope H, David A, Pelosi A, Mann A. Predictors of chronic "postviral" fatigue. Lancet 344:864–868, 1994.

39. Kiecolt Glaser JK, Fisher LD, et al. Marital quality, marital disruption, and immune function. Psychosom Med 49:13–34, 1987.

CHAPTER SIX

The Fatigue Workup

A comprehensive workup is essential to diagnosing fatigue and choosing an effective course of management. The workup includes the patient and family history, physical examination, and laboratory testing (Table 6-1). There are also specialized studies that can be performed for the diagnosis of specific diseases.

HISTORY AND PHYSICAL EXAMINATION

The history should include both a comprehensive personal and family history. The physician should prepare to invest substantial time in the history,

Table 6-1. Elements of the General Workup for Fatigue

Element	Goal(s)
Personal history	Identify a specific disease that may be the cause of fatigue
	Distinguish between "normal" and "pathologic" fatigue
	Identify fatigue severity, chronicity, triggers, and variations
	Assess sleep patterns and medication use
	Observe patient for signs of negative affect/mood disorders
	Assess for history of substance abuse
	Assess for history of physical/emotional abuse or other chronic stressors
Family history	Assess for history of affective/mood disorders
	Assess family history of alcoholism/substance abuse
Physical examination	Vital sign assessment
	HEENT (head, ear, eye, nose, and throat) evaluation to check for lymph node enlargement, thyroid enlargement, and signs of infection
	Chest exam to detect breathing/cardiac abnormalities
	Neurologic examination to detect abnormalities of affect, mental status, and motor/sensory function
	Rheumatologic examination for synovitis/trigger points
	Skin assessment for evidence of bites/rash

(continued)

Table 6-1. Cont'd.

Element	Goal(s)
	Abdominal assessment for hepatosplenomegaly
Laboratory testing	See Table 6-2
Specialized studies	Sleep clinic referral to rule out idiopathic sleep disorders, sleep apnea, movement disorders during sleep
	Breathing tests (e.g., spirometry) to rule out chronic obstructive pulmonary disease
	Neuromuscular testing for suspected peripheral muscular fatigue

especially if it is the initial history taking. Because fatigue symptoms rarely occur alone, the goals of the history and physical examination should be to inquire about other symptoms or signs that may suggest a specific disease, and to gain as full an understanding of the patient as possible, from both a physical and psychological standpoint.

The physician should distinguish between pathologic fatigue (an overwhelming sense of tiredness or loss of energy that persists after rest) versus normal, transient, mild fatigue or symptoms of daytime sleepiness. The Epworth Sleepiness Scale (discussed in Chapter 4) can be used to assess excessive daytime sleepiness and the presence of an idiopathic sleep disorder such as narcolepsy.

Specific questions about fatigue should include its initial onset (acute or chronic), whether there are any variations during the day or night, the severity of the fatigue (which can be assessed using a fatigue scale) and whether the patient can identify any triggering factors that may worsen fatigue (such as heat, exercise, or personal or family stress) or situations and activities that can ameliorate fatigue (e.g., whether fatigue improves after exercise, after hearing unexpected good news, or after resting).

The history should include an assessment of professional activities and activities of daily living. The physician should inquire about the patient's occupation and level of stress at work, as well as any changes in occupational, educational, social, or personal activities.

The physician should ask whether the patient has been diagnosed with any specific disorders that may be associated with fatigue. Prominent disorders in which fatigue is a symptom include malignancy, Parkinson's disease, chronic fatigue syndrome or fibromyalgia, multiple sclerosis, Lyme disease, hypothyroidism, metabolic diseases, epilepsy, chronic obstructive pulmonary disease (COPD), obstructive sleep apnea, infectious hepatitis, systemic lupus erythematosus, rheumatoid arthritis, and congestive heart failure. The physician should also ask about a history of recent surgery or traumatic events.

Nighttime sleep patterns should be assessed during the history. The patient's bed partner can be instrumental in identifying factors that interfere with normal sleep, such as restless legs syndrome, periodic limb movements, or sleep apneas/hypopneas.

The individual's medication history should indicate whether the person uses any medications that may potentially induce tiredness or fatigue, such as benzodiazepines, muscle relaxants, antihistamines, and sedatives. Recent additions of medications or changes in dose/dosage schedules should be assessed.

The physician should ask about the patient's history of infection/fever, as recent viral infections (e.g., influenza) can induce fatigue symptoms. Because of the association between human immunodeficiency virus (HIV) and fatigue, HIV testing should be encouraged in any person at risk. Similarly, those at potential risk for Lyme disease (e.g., those in suburban or rural areas, especially in the Northeast) should be asked about a history of tick/insect bites, expanding rash, or joint swelling.

Lifestyle history can include questions about relationships with family members because stress and/or depression may be associated with "dysfunctional" family situations. Smoking history should be assessed because respiratory disorders such as COPD may lead to fatigue. Caffeine intake should be determined because excessive consumption may interfere with sleep patterns.

During the interview, the physician should observe the patient carefully for signs of negative affect that may be indicative of depression. The psychological history taking can be challenging. Patients may not be aware of depressive/fatigue symptoms, or they may have accepted them as a normal part of their lives. Patients may not be willing to admit potential psychological problems, and may be quite adamant that their fatigue be attributable to physical and not psychological factors (as in the case of somatization disorders). The physician should focus on the potential presence of depression or anxiety disorders; recent weight loss or gain, loss of appetite, feelings of sadness, or recent loss of interest in activities are all signs of depression.

The psychological history should include questions about the patient's experience with alcohol or other drugs of abuse, prescription medication abuse, and a history of spousal abuse. If any of these are suspected, a psychiatric consultation is appropriate.

The person's family history should include the presence of major depression, anxiety disorders, or affective disorders, and alcoholism/substance abuse. It is appropriate for the physician to ask about a history of heart disease, metabolic disease such as diabetes or hypothyroidism, and cancer.

PHYSICAL
EXAMINATION/LABORATORY TESTING

A comprehensive physical exam should include temperature assessment, a HEENT evaluation to check for signs of lymph node enlargement, thyroid size, throat and ear redness or swelling, or otitis. During the chest examination the physician should check for the presence of abnormal heart and lung sounds that may indicate the need for cardiac/pulmonary testing. The skin should be examined carefully for evidence of bites or rash, and the abdomen should be palpated and assessed for hepatosplenomegaly.

A thorough neurologic examination is an integral part of the physical examination in the fatigued patient. Abnormalities of affect, mental status, motor and sensory function, balance and muscle changes of atrophy or weakness need be checked. A rheumatologic assessment for trigger points and synovitis should be included. A number of laboratory tests are available to help determine the underlying cause of fatigue and to rule out potential diseases. A nonexhaustive list of laboratory tests is shown in Table 6-2.[1] Routine laboratory tests should be used to exclude causes of fatigue such as infection and metabolic disease. Of note, immune assays, such as viral titers to Epstein-Barr virus, are not recommended in the workup of the fatigued patient.[2]

Table 6-2. Laboratory Tests that are Useful in the Fatigue Workup

Test	Assesses for
Serial morning or afternoon temperatures	Infection, malignancy
Complete blood cell count and differential	Infection, malignancy
Erythrocyte sedimentation rate	Abscess, osteomyelitis, endocarditis, cancer, tuberculosis, mycosis, collagen-vascular disease
Electrolytes	Adrenal insufficiency, tuberculosis
Glucose	Diabetes mellitus
Blood urea nitrogen/ creatinine	Renal failure
Calcium	Hyperparathyroidism, cancer, sarcoidosis
Total bilirubin	Hepatitis, hemolysis
Serum glutamic oxalocetic transaminase (SGOT)	Hepatocellular disease
Serum glutamic pyruvic transaminase (SGPT)	Hepatocellular abscess
Alkaline phosphatase	Obstructive liver disease
Creatine phosphokinase (CPK)	Muscle disease
Urinalysis	Renal disease, proteinuria
Posteroanterior lateral chest radiograph	Cardiopulmonary disease
Antinuclear antibodies	Systemic lupus erythematosus, other collagen-vascular disease
Thyroid-stimulating hormone	Hypothyroidism
HIV antibody test	HIV/AIDS

(continued)

Table 6-2. Cont'd

Test	Assesses for
Purified protein derivative	Tuberculosis
Hepatitis screen	Hepatitis
Lyme serologies	Lyme disease/post-Lyme syndrome

(Source: Adapted from Morrison RE, Keating HJ. Fatigue in primary care. Obstet Gynecol Clin North Am 28:225–235, 2001.)

Assessments of fatigue and mood at baseline and at follow-up can help assess changes or response to interventions. If the history-taking indicates the possibility of a sleep disorder, the patient may be referred to a sleep clinic to rule out idiopathic sleep disorders, obstructive sleep apnea, or movement disorders that interfere with the sleep cycle. Specialized breathing tests include spirometry to rule out COPD. In cases of suspected peripheral muscular fatigue, neurologic referral and neuromuscular testing can be performed.

CONCLUSIONS

The fatigue workup should be designed to determine the potential causes and severity of fatigue and systematically rule out potential causes, including neurologic, cardiac, infectious, metabolic, and neoplastic disease. Careful attention to the psychological history-taking is especially appropriate to identify affective disorders that may lead to depression. As with any workup, the physician should use his or her best judgment in the workup for fatigue, ordering appropriate laboratory tests and specialized testing when necessary.

REFERENCES

1. Morrison RE, Keating HJ. Fatigue in primary care. Obstet Gynecol Clin North Am 28:225–237, 2001.
2. Fukuda K, Straus SE, Hickie I, et al. The chronic fatigue syndrome: a comprehensive approach to its definition and study. Ann Intern Med 121:953–959, 1994.

PART TWO

Fatigue in Specific Disorders

CHAPTER SEVEN

Multiple Sclerosis–Related Fatigue

Much of what has been learned about fatigue in neurologic illness has stemmed from work in multiple sclerosis (MS). Although the motor symptoms of MS (e.g., tremor and spasticity) are more visible to observers, fatigue has been consistently reported as extremely troublesome to the patient. Its frequency has been reported to be as high as 97%, and many patients consider it to be the worst symptom of their disease.[1] It can have profound negative effects, impairing quality of life, concentration, and memory.[2] It also has emotional consequences that include anxiety, depression, and irritability.[1]

Identifying and managing fatigue in the MS patient is a challenge because there are few consistent predictors of this symptom. MS–related fatigue does not correlate well with neuropsychological outcomes[3] or the level of disease activity on magnetic resonance imaging. It correlates either weakly or not at all with the duration of disease, the patient's disability level on the Expanded Disability Status Scale (EDSS), or the clinical MS subtype (relapsing-remitting, secondary progressive, or primary progressive).[4,5]

PATHOGENESIS

The pathogenesis of fatigue remains uncertain. Some have suggested that demyelination of axons is the central cause for MS fatigue. Others suggest that specific regions such as the basal ganglia, hypothalamus, or brain-stem areas are responsible for decreased arousal, motivation, and motor readiness, which lead to fatigue. However no one anatomic site within the central nervous system has been identified that explains fatigue.[1,5–7]

There is a long list of demographic and other variables that show little to no association with fatigue. For example, neither age nor gender has shown a meaningful correlation with fatigue. Similarly, perceived fatigue does not show an association with performance on conventional neuropsychological tests[3,8] or tasks of motor function.

Medications found to ameliorate fatigue have shown inconsistent effects on cognitive function,[3,9] and changes in cognitive function across a test session are not correlated with changes in perceived fatigue.[2,10]

Sleep studies also have failed to demonstrate a consistent association with MS fatigue.[11] The failure to identify laboratory or physiologic markers of fatigue has limited our understanding of this major symptom.

Immune factors may contribute to fatigue. Medications such as interferon-α and interferon-β[12,13] produce prominent fatigue as an initial side effect. An association between perceived fatigue was noted in a study that measured circulating immune activation,[14] although others examining inflammatory cytokines and fatigue have not replicated these findings.[15] Given the sensitivity of circulating inflammatory cytokines to many variables, and the difficulties in their measurement, one can imagine that an association of this biologic marker with such a heterogeneous entity as fatigue would be difficult to consistently detect.

It seems reasonable to speculate that fatigue has a neuronal basis. The strongest support to date comes from studies of altered cerebral metabolism. Positron emission tomography in subjects with MS identified a significant association between perceived fatigue as measured by the Fatigue Severity Scale (FSS) and cerebral glucose availability.[16,17] Disruption in neurotransmitter systems may underlie fatigue.[18] An association between perceived fatigue and changes in the amplitude of event-related and motor-related evoked potentials has been seen, but these studies have involved only a small number of patients and some potential confounding factors were not fully controlled for.[6,19,20]

Presently, there is little evidence that changes in central motor conduction are associated with perceived MS fatigue.[6,19,21,22] However, intermittent use-dependent block of central conduction could partially account for the observed benefit of fatigue with cooling or 3, 4-aminopyridine treatment. Studies demonstrating abnormal muscle metabolism in MS are also of interest, but do not fully explain the subjective experience of fatigue.[23] Research designed to examine physiologic changes in conjunction with definition of subjective states is perhaps the most promising direction for future studies.[17]

DIAGNOSIS

Unlike most disease areas, there is a set of published guidelines for fatigue in MS.[24] These guidelines, published in 1998 by the MS Council for Clinical

Practice Guidelines, are available on the World Wide Web at www.pva.org. They were formulated by a multidisciplinary team including neurologists, rehabilitation specialists, nurses, social workers, and psychological care providers. In the guidelines, fatigue is defined as "a subjective lack of physical and/or mental energy that is perceived by the individual or caregiver to interfere with usual and desired activities."[24] Fatigue is characterized as either acute (a new or significant increase in feelings of fatigue in the previous 6 weeks) or chronic persistent (present for any amount of time on 50% of the days for more than 6 weeks). Under either definition, the guidelines emphasize that fatigue limits functional activities and quality of life.

Numerous factors can cause or contribute to fatigue in the MS patient, including environmental surroundings, physical health, the presence of a sleep disorder, or mental health problems (Table 7-1).[24] In diagnosing fatigue, the physician should determine the presence of any secondary causes, such as medication use. A number of drugs can cause symptoms of fatigue in the MS patient, including the interferon betas, which are used to reduce the incidence of disease exacerbations (Table 7-2).[24] Medications such as baclofen or tizanidine, which are used to treat spasticity, can also cause feelings of tiredness or weakness, and can exacerbate existing fatigue symptoms.

Table 7-1. Potential Contributors to MS–Related Fatigue

Primary disease-related processes (e.g., demyelination, axonal destruction, inflammation, brain hypometabolism)

Disability or deconditioning

Pain

Comorbid conditions

Medications

Iatrogenic conditions

Sleep disorders (primary or secondary)

Psychological factors (anxiety, depression stress, other psychological conditions)

Environmental factors (physical, social, cultural)

(Reprinted with permission from the Multiple Sclerosis Council for Clinical Practice Guidelines. Fatigue and Multiple Sclerosis. Washington, DC: Paralyzed Veterans Association, 1998.)

Introduction of a new medication that may cause fatigue should be considered in the evaluation of new onset fatigue.

In diagnosing MS–related fatigue, the focus should be primarily on the patient's perceived fatigue level. The complaints of patients with MS–related fatigue often involve depressed energy, malaise, rapid decreases in strength with continued activity, and difficulty in concentration and performance of tasks that require mental effort. Because patients may not voluntarily report these deficits (or even be aware of them), it is important to use questions designed specifically to elicit this information.

Table 7-2. Classes of Agents that May Cause or Exacerbate MS–Related Fatigue

The following classes of agents are often prescribed for MS patients. Fatigue may be common in one or more of the agents in these classes. Check the prescribing information of any individual agent in these classes that you may prescribe.

Analgesics
Anticonvulsants
Antidepressants
Antihistamines
Antihypertensives/cardiac medications
Anti-inflammatories
Antipsychotics
Asthma drugs
Carbonic anhydrase inhibitors
Diabetic agents
Gastrointestinal agents
Genitourinary agents
Hormone replacement therapies
Immune modulators
Muscle relaxants
Nicotine agents
Sedatives/hypnotics

(Reprinted with permission from Multiple Sclerosis Council for Clinical Practice Guidelines. Fatigue and Multiple Sclerosis. Washington, DC: Paralyzed Veterans Association, 1998.)

Fatigue can be assessed using one of the self-reporting scales outlined in Chapter 3, such as the FSS. A score of *equal to or greater than* 4 on the FSS is generally indicative of severe fatigue.[25] The

MS–Specific Fatigue Scale (MS–FS) has been designed to ask about factors specific to MS–related fatigue, such as the effects of heat.[26] The use of this scale, however, has not been shown to be more advantageous than the use of more general fatigue scales. Self-reporting scales are easily administered at each visit, and can be used to gauge the patient's response to treatment. In cases of localized muscle fatigue, the diagnosis can be made using measures of force generation and recovery time.[27]

TREATMENT

A comprehensive treatment plan for fatigue is discussed in more detail in Chapter 17. As in other diseases, fatigue in the MS patient should involve a broad-based, multidisciplinary approach. Because respiratory deconditioning and muscle disuse can contribute significantly to fatigue symptoms,[28] attempts should be made to increase strength and mobility. It was once believed that MS patients should not engage in exercise, in order to conserve strength; however, an exercise program that is appropriately tailored to the patient's level of ability will ultimately improve strength, mobility, and flexibility.[29] Because exercise may increase the risk of overheating, measures such as the use of cooling garments can be taken to reduce this risk in patients who are heat sensitive.

Although several studies have documented the exacerbation of symptoms in response to thermal stress, these studies utilized unreliable techniques to measure core temperature and those studies employing more efficacious techniques failed to support these findings.[30] In addition, Mostert[31] found only 6% of the patients studied had an increase in their fatigue symptomology following a 4-week exercise program.

Studies examining exercise as an intervention for fatigue and as a means to increase patient activity levels and physical functioning have reported on its benefits for patients' self-reported health perception, physical activity patterns, perceived general health, and fatigue.[31,32] In addition, improvements in cardiorespiratory fitness and skeletal muscle functioning have been realized following short-term exercise programs.[30]

Two factors are paramount when developing exercise programs for any patient, including those with MS. The first is tailoring the exercise regimen to meet the functional abilities of each patient. The second is the context in which the clinician "sells" the patient on the efficacy of this intervention and in incorporating techniques designed to increase patient compliance.

Developing exercise programs to meet the individual needs of MS patients must take into account several factors. Examination of baseline activity patterns, functional ability, and physical limitations due to disease is needed to develop a program that will activate working muscles, but avoid overloading the individual.[33] In addition, the patient's cardiorespiratory fitness should be measured, as MS patients with moderate disease impairment may have deficits in this area.[30] A hierarchical program that is designed to meet the individual needs of the patient should then be developed, with patients progressing through the different stages (passive range of motion, active resistance, specific strengthening, integrated strength exercises, and increases in the amount of time devoted to cardiovascular workouts) at their own pace.[33]

When initially presenting patients with these programs, which tend to have a low rate of compliance, the same importance and weight given when prescribing pharmacologic treatments should be applied. The physician should expound on the efficacy and benefits of the program and present it as a structured regimen, with explicit details as to the number of days each exercise is performed, the amount of time spent on each exercise, and the specific number of repetitions performed. Cognitive behavioral interventions, tailored to provide the patient with rewards that are meaningful to them and that would motivate them to complete the exercise program developed, should also be employed. Token economies (i.e., offering acknowledgment or a reward for achieving goals), involving significant others in monitoring compliance, and providing encouragement and keeping a diary of exercise activities to be presented at follow-up visits are all methods that can aid in increasing patient adherence to an exercise program.

PHARMACOLOGIC THERAPIES

There is no drug currently approved by the US Food and Drug Administration for the treatment of primary MS–related fatigue. However, a number of agents have been used successfully over the past two decades (Table 7-3):

Amantadine: Amantadine is an antiviral agent that most likely exerts its positive effects on MS–related fatigue through dopaminergic mechanisms. It has been studied in several small, randomized, clinical trials, and appears to offer favorable results in approximately one third of patients with mild fatigue.[26,34–36] It has the advantage of being inexpensive, and has a

Table 7-3. Medications Most Commonly Used for MS Fatigue

Drug	Starting Dose	Usual Maintenance Dose	Usual Maximum Dose	Adverse Effects
Amantadine	100 mg q AM or 100 mg bid	100 mg bid	300 mg/d	Livedo reticularis, insomnia
Modafinil	100 mg q AM	200 mg q AM or 100 mg bid	400 mg/d	Headache, insomnia
Pemoline	18.75 mg/d	18.75–55.5 mg/d	93.75 mg/d	Irritability, restlessness, insomnia(?), LFT changes

good side-effect profile: Some of the most common adverse effects are insomnia, dizziness, and vivid dreams. Dosing can be started at 100 mg bid. There have been anecdotal reports of a loss of efficacy with long-term use of amantadine; if this occurs, the patient may benefit from a temporary "drug holiday."

Pemoline: The central nervous system (CNS) stimulant pemoline has also been used for the treatment of MS–related fatigue. Results with this medication have been mixed at best, with clinical trials tending to show efficacy only at higher doses (e.g., 75 mg/day).[26,37] The adverse effects of pemoline are consistent with those of other CNS stimulants, and include increased motor activity, irritability, and insomnia. This drug has also received a "black box" warning by the US Food and Drug Administration, based on several reports of liver failure.[38] Its performance in clinical studies and its adverse-effect profile suggest that it should not be used as a first-line option for MS–related fatigue. However, because patients' responses to fatigue medications vary substantially, some patients may respond well to it.

Modafinil: Modafinil is a wake-promoting agent that is approved for the treatment of excessive daytime sleepiness associated with narcolepsy.

It has a different mechanism of action than CNS stimulants. Instead of the global cortical activation of stimulant medications, modafinil is believed to act along pathways of "normal wakefulness," increasing cortical activity in the frontal lobe by activation of histaminergic pathways from the tuberomammillary nucleus.[39] As a result, it does not cause the global CNS activation of the CNS stimulants, and its abuse potential is lower.

A recently published clinical trial of patients whose fatigue was considered severe (FSS scores of >4) showed good efficacy for this agent, with a significant decrease in fatigue scores on the FSS, Modified Fatigue Impact Scale, and Visual Analog Scale for Fatigue compared with base-line (Figure 7-1).[40] Modafinil has been the only drug to move scores on the FSS significantly compared with placebo.

The dose used in this study was 200 mg; a higher dose of 400 mg did not have a significant effect on fatigue, although it did improve excessive daytime sleepiness scores consistent with studies in narcolepsy populations.[41] Based on its efficacy, modafinil should be considered a first-line therapy in patients with moderate to severe fatigue, and can also be used as a second-line agent in patients who do

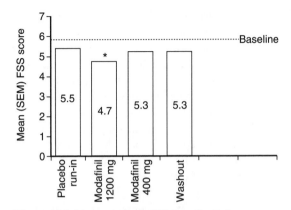

Figure 7-1. Mean scores (±SEM) on the Fatigue Severity Scale (FSS) at the end of each treatment phase for modafinil. The dashed line represents the mean score at the baseline visit. (Reprinted with permission from Rammohan KW, Rosenberg JH, Lynn DJ, et al. Efficacy and safety of modafinil [Provigil] for the treatment of fatigue in multiple sclerosis: a two-centre phase 2 study. J Neurol Neurosurg Psychiatry 72:179–183, 2002.)

not respond to amantadine. Dosing can begin at 100 mg/day and be titrated up to 200 mg either once daily or in divided doses in the morning and early afternoon. It is well tolerated: The most common adverse effect is headache in approximately 15% to 20% of patients, which should subside as the patient becomes accustomed to the medication.

Other Medications: Other possible treatment options for MS–related fatigue include the use of activating antidepressants such as bupropion, venlafaxine, and fluoxetine. Because of the association between fatigue and depression, treatment of depression in patients who are indeed depressed may help to reduce symptoms of fatigue. The published evidence on the use of these medications specifically for fatigue symptoms is limited.[42] However, because there are anecdotal reports of efficacy, their use should be considered.

The aminopyridines have been cited as another potentially effective class of medications. Although they have been shown to improve ease of transferring and ambulation in MS patients, they are not recommended for use in MS–related fatigue.[43,44]

CONCLUSIONS

While MS–related fatigue remains poorly understood, its impact on the patient should not be underestimated. Unfortunately, most physicians still do not assess MS patients for fatigue.[45]

MS–Related Fatigue: Key Concepts

- Fatigue is present in the large majority of MS patients, and is the single worst symptom of the disease in many patients. It is important to identify because it can have profound impacts on daily functioning, quality of life, and employment.

- Fatigue is most likely a central phenomenon related to the demyelination of neurons and destruction of axons in the central nervous system. Nerve conduction difficulties can also cause peripheral muscle fatigue.

- All MS patients should be evaluated for fatigue because it occurs independent of disease subtype, age, gender, or level of disability. Diagnosis focuses on the patient's perceived fatigue severity as measured on self-report scales such as the FSS.

- The treatment of fatigue must focus on maintaining and improving conditioning through an exercise program. Both aerobic conditioning and strength-building exercises should be incorporated into the plan.

- The antiviral drug amantadine and the wake-promoting drug modafinil have both shown significant benefit in reducing fatigue severity in MS patients. If secondary causes of fatigue are controlled and fatigue persists, pharmacologic therapy should be used.

Treatment with both nonpharmacologic and pharmacologic therapies has proven beneficial, and can help to restore energy levels, mobility, and psychological well being.

REFERENCES

1. Bakshi R, Shaikh ZA, Miletich RS, et al. Fatigue in multiple sclerosis and its relationship to depression and neurologic disability. Mult Scler 6:181–185, 2000.
2. Krupp LB, Elkins LE. Fatigue and declines in cognitive functioning in multiple sclerosis. Neurology 55:934–939, 2000.
3. Geisler MS, Sliwinski M, Coyle PK, et al. The effects of amantadine and pemoline on cognitive functioning in multiple sclerosis. Arch Neurol 53:185–188, 1996.
4. Bakshi R, Miletich RS, Hanschel K, et al. Fatigue in multiple sclerosis: cross-sectional correlation with brain MRI findings in 71 patients. Neurology 53:1151–1153, 1999.
5. Mainero C, Faroni J, Gasperini C, et al. Fatigue and magnetic resonance imaging activity in multiple sclerosis. J Neurol 246:454–458, 1999.
6. Colombo B, Martinelli Boneschi F, Rossi P, et al. MRI and motor evoked potential findings in non-disabled multiple sclerosis patients with and without symptoms of fatigue. J Neurol 247:506–509, 2000.
7. van der Werf SP, Jongen PJ, Lycklama a Nijeholt GJ, et al. Fatigue in multiple sclerosis: interrelations

between fatigue complaints, cerebral MRI abnormalities and neurological disability. J Neurol Sci 160:164–170, 1998.

8. Schwartz CE, Coulthard-Morris L, Zeng Q. Psychosocial correlates of fatigue in multiple sclerosis. Arch Phys Med Rehabil 77:165–170, 1996.

9. Sailer M, Heinze HJ, Schoenfeld MA, et al. Amantadine influences cognitive processing in patients with multiple sclerosis. Pharmacopsychiatry 33:28–37, 2000.

10. Paul RH, Beatty WW, Schneider R, et al. Cognitive and physical fatigue in multiple sclerosis: relations between self-report and objective performance. Appl Neuropsych 5:143–148, 1998.

11. Bohr KC, Haas J. Sleep related breathing disorders do not explain daytime fatigue in multiple sclerosis. Mult Scler 4:289a, 1998.

12. Quesada JR, Talpax M, Rios A, et al. Clinical toxicity of interferons in cancer patients, a review. J Clin Oncol 4:234–243, 1986.

13. Neilly LK, Goodin DS, Goodkin DE, Hause SL. Side effect profile of interferon beta-1b in MS: results of an open label trial. Neurology 46:552–554, 1996.

14. Iriarte J, Subira ML, Castro P. Modalities of fatigue in multiple sclerosis: correlation with clinical and biological factors. Mult Scler 6:124–130, 2000.

15. Giovannoni G, Thompson AJ, Miller DH, Thompson EJ. Fatigue is not associated with raised inflammatory markers in multiple sclerosis. Neurology 57:676–681, 2001.

16. Roelcke U, Kappos L, Lechner-Scott J, et al. Reduced glucose metabolism in the frontal cortex and basal ganglia of multiple sclerosis patients with fatigue: a

18F-fluorodeoxyglucose positron emission tomography study. Neurology 48:1566–1571, 1997.

17. Filippi M, Rocca MA, Colombo B, et al. Functional magnetic resonance imaging correlates of fatigue in multiple sclerosis. Neuroimage 15:559–567, 2002.

18. Heilman KM, Watson RT. Fatigue. Neurology Network Commentary 1:283–287, 1997.

19. Sandroni P, Walker C, Starr A. Fatigue in patients with multiple sclerosis; motor pathway conduction and event-related potentials. Arch Neurol 49:517–524, 1992.

20. Brasil-Neto JP, Cohen LG, Hallet M. Central fatigue as revealed by postexercise decrement of motor evoked potentials. Muscle Nerve 17:713–719, 1994.

21. Comi G, Leocani L, Rossi P, Colombo B. Physiopathology and treatment of fatigue in multiple sclerosis. J Neurol 248:174–179, 2001.

22. Sheean GL, Murray MF, Rothwell SG. An electrophysiologic study of the mechanism of fatigue in MS. Brain 120:299–316, 1997.

23. Sharma KR, Kent-Braun J, Mynhier MA, et al. Evidence of abnormal intramuscular component of fatigue in multiple sclerosis. Muscle Nerve 18:1403–1411, 1995.

24. Multiple Sclerosis Council for Clinical Practice Guidelines. Fatigue and Multiple Sclerosis. Washington, DC: Paralyzed Veterans Association, 1998.

25. Krupp LB, LaRocca NG, Muir-Nash J, Steinberg AD. The fatigue severity scale: application to patients with multiple sclerosis and systemic lupus erythematosus. Arch Neurol 46:1121–1123, 1989.

26. Krupp LB, Coyle PK, Doscher C, et al. Fatigue therapy in multiple sclerosis: results of a double-blind,

randomized, parallel trial of amantadine, pemoline, and placebo. Neurology 45:1956–1961, 1995.

27. Schwid SR, Thornton CA, Pandya S, et al. Quantitative assessment of motor fatigue and strength in MS. Neurology 53:743–750, 1999.

28. Kent-Braun JA, Sharma KR, Weiner MW, Miller RG. Effects of exercise on muscle activation and metabolism in multiple sclerosis. Muscle Nerve 17:1162–1169, 1994.

29. Petajan JH, Gappmaier E, White AT, et al. Impact of aerobic training on fitness and quality of life in multiple sclerosis. Ann Neurol 39:432–441, 1996.

30. Ponichtera-Mulcare JA. Exercise and multiple sclerosis. Med Sci Sports Exercise 25:451–465, 1993.

31. Mostert S, Kesselring J. Effects of a short-term exercise program on aerobic fitness, fatigue, health perception and activity level of subjects with multiple sclerosis. Mult Scler 8:161–168, 2002.

32. Stuifbergen AK. Physical activity and perceived health status in persons with multiple sclerosis. J Neurosci Nursing 29:238–243, 1997.

33. Petajan JH, White AT. Recommendations for physical activity in patients with multiple sclerosis. Sports Medicine 27:179–191, 1999.

34. Murray TJ. Amantadine therapy for fatigue in multiple sclerosis. Can J Neurol Sci 12:251–254, 1985.

35. Canadian MS Research Group. A randomized controlled trial of amantadine in fatigue associated with MS. Can J Neurosci 14:273–279, 1987.

36. Cohen RA, Fisher M. Amantadine treatment of fatigue associated with multiple sclerosis. Arch Neurol 46:676–680, 1989.

37. Weinshenker BG, Penman M, Bass B, et al. A double-blind, randomized, crossover trial of

pemoline in fatigue associated with multiple sclerosis. Neurology 42:1468–1471, 1992.

38. Cylert (pemoline) package insert. Chicago: Abbott Laboratories, June 1999.

39. Scammell TE, Estabrooke IV, McCarthy MT, et al. Hypothalamic arousal regions are activated during modafinil-induced wakefulness. J Neurosci 20:8620–8628, 2000.

40. Rammohan KW, Rosenberg JH, Lynn DJ, et al. Efficacy and safety of modafinil (Provigil) for the treatment of fatigue in multiple sclerosis: a two-centre phase 2 study. J Neurol Neurosurg Psychiatry 72:179–183, 2002.

41. Randomized trial of modafinil as a treatment for the excessive daytime somnolence of narcolepsy: US Modafinil in Narcolepsy Multicenter Study Group. Neurology 54:1166–1175, 2000.

42. Duffy JC, Campbell J. Bupropion for the treatment of fatigue associated with multiple sclerosis. Psychosomatics 35:170–171, 1994.

43. Polman CH, Bertelsmann FW, van Loenen AC, Koetsier JC. 4-aminopyridine in the treatment of patients with multiple sclerosis: long-term efficacy and safety. Arch Neurol 51(3):292–296, 1994.

44. Bever CT. The current status of studies of aminopyridines in multiple sclerosis. Ann Neurol 36(suppl 1):S118–S121, 1994.

45. Tremlett HL, Luscombe DK, Wiles CM. Prescribing for multiple sclerosis patients in general practice: a case-control study. J Clin Pharm Ther 26:437–444, 2001.

Fatigue in Postpolio Syndrome

The term *postpolio syndrome* refers to the late development of neuromuscular symptoms, including fatigue, new weakness, and pain, in patients who have recovered from acute paralytic poliomyelitis.[1,2] It is estimated that there are more than 1.5 million polio survivors in the United States, and that approximately one third to one half of them will develop postpolio syndrome.[3,4] Generally, symptoms such as fatigue appear 3 to 4 decades after the acute phase of illness, and are very slowly progressive.[3] The frequency of fatigue in those with postpolio syndrome is high: In a Norwegian study of nearly 1500 polio survivors, nearly 80% experienced fatigue during exercise, and nearly 60% experienced a form of general fatigue.[5]

CAUSES OF FATIGUE IN POSTPOLIO SYNDROME

The cause of fatigue in postpolio syndrome is unclear. It is unlikely that fatigue is to the result of persistent poliovirus infection or an immune-mediated process.[3] As with other neurologic diseases, central, peripheral, and chronic illness–related causes have been offered.

Certain brain studies have supported the theory that postpolio syndrome is a centrally related phenomenon. Postmortem studies have examined the presence of polio-induced lesions in the brain and their potential relationship to postpolio symptoms, including fatigue. Histopathologic examination in 158 individuals who contracted polio before 1950 found damage to the reticular activating system and monoaminergic neurons in the brain. The damage is believed to be implicated in postpolio syndrome fatigue.[6]

Also supporting a centrally mediated disease mechanism is the fact that sleep disorders appear to play at least a partial role in postpolio syndrome fatigue. More than half of postpolio syndrome patients have reported that they have abnormal movements during sleep, possibly related to poliovirus-induced damage to the brain and spinal cord that affect their sleep cycle. These movements include generalized random myoclonus, periodic limb movements of sleep, and restless legs syndrome.[7]

Central nervous system factors may also result in cognitive fatigue, which appears to be a significant concern in postpolio syndrome patients, especially those with more severe fatigue. In a study of six polio survivors who were given a battery of neuropsychological tests, those with severe fatigue demonstrated clinically significant deficits in attention, concentration, and information processing speed. (No impairments were seen in verbal memory.)[8]

Peripherally, one of the prevailing theories is that the fatigue experienced by postpolio syndrome patients is an augmented form of peripheral muscular fatigue.[9] This may be related to premature exhaustion of the motor neurons that develop after acute poliomyelitis.[3]

Factors associated with chronic illness may play important roles in postpolio syndrome. Emotional stress may be a trigger for postpolio syndrome fatigue. The involvement of the stress response from activation of the hypothalamic-pituitary-adrenal axis, as well as common findings of deficits in attention, has led some researchers to theorize that postpolio syndrome fatigue and chronic fatigue syndrome have a common pathophysiology.[10] In addition, deconditioning due to low activity level is an obvious problem for a large percentage of polio survivors; thus, reduced aerobic capacity may be a contributor to fatigue and general tiredness.[9]

Studies of psychological correlates in postpolio syndrome fatigue suggest that psychological factors do not appear to play a significant role in the development of muscle weakness and accompanying symptoms such as fatigue. In a study of 24 patients evaluated using various personality inventories and fatigue scales, there was no relationship between depression, anxiety, or other psychopathologies and postpolio syndrome.[1] However, low levels of social support have been correlated with self-reported fatigue on the Fatigue Severity Scale (FSS).[11]

There do appear to be some predictive factors for postpolio syndrome fatigue, including greater age at time to clinical presentation of the syndrome and a longer time since acute polio infection. Factors such as weight gain, muscle pain with exercise, and joint pain, are associated with fatigue and muscle weakness.[2] Age at the time of acute polio infection, physical activity level, the degree of recovery after polio, and gender do not appear to be predictive of postpolio syndrome fatigue.[2]

Importantly, the appearance of postpolio syndrome fatigue may not be limited to patients with a history of acute paralytic polio. Some data have suggested that nonparalytic polio, or *abortive polio,* in which the poliovirus does not appear to enter the central nervous system or damage neurons, may also be associated with late-onset fatigue.[12]

The degree of fatigue in postpolio syndrome appears to be moderate to severe. In one study of 12 subjects with postpolio syndrome, the average score on the FSS was between 4 and 5. Fatigue peaked in the late morning or early afternoon.[13] In addition, the disease course does not appear to be drastically progressive, and the degree of impairment related to fatigue is generally limited.[14]

MANAGEMENT CONSIDERATIONS

It is important for the physician to ask specifically about a history of poliovirus infection, especially in the elderly patient who may have been a child before the introduction of polio vaccinations. Because the development of postpolio syndrome, and its accompanying fatigue, can take decades to manifest, the association between acute polio infection and postpolio syndrome may not be obvious. Fatigue accompanied by muscular weakness and joint muscle pain, along with neuropathic electromyography changes, are clues to the presence of postpolio syndrome.[9]

A number of options have been proposed for the management of fatigue in postpolio syndrome. For individual muscle weakness, a case study has shown that high-intensity, short duration muscle strengthening exercise can increase objective measures of muscle strength, as well as subjective feelings of strength.[15] However, the long-term effects of exercise have not been sufficiently evaluated.[3]

There is support for the use of rest and energy conservation strategies, as well as strategies to simplify work skills, to manage the fatigue of postpolio syndrome.[13] Given the potential association between stress and postpolio fatigue, strategies to minimize both physical and emotional stress should be employed. Use of orthoses, mobility aids, or adaptive equipment can also be helpful.[16]

Several drug treatments have been explored for fatigue in postpolio syndrome. The dopamine-agonist bromocriptine was used in a small trial of five survivors of paralytic polio who continued to report moderate to severe fatigue following more conservative treatments. Bromocriptine in a dose of 12.5 mg/day resulted in self-reported symptom improvement in three patients. Difficulties in attention, concentration, and fatigue on awakening were also decreased.[17]

Based on the efficacy of amantadine in multiple sclerosis, another group of researchers conducted

Postpolio Syndrome: Key Concepts

- Up to 80% of persons with postpolio syndrome experience some form of fatigue. Postpolio syndrome with its accompanying fatigue can take 3 to 4 decades to develop after acute polio infection.

- Postpolio syndrome may be a disease of the central nervous system (as suggested by the presence of cognitive difficulties and sleep disorders) or the peripheral nervous system (related to premature exhaustion of the motor neurons that develop after acute infection).

- Factors related to chronic illness, including stress-related endocrine dysfunction, may also be a cause of postpolio syndrome.

- It is important to be aware of the possibility of postpolio syndrome, especially in the elderly patient who was alive before the development of polio vaccines. Given the length of time that postpolio syndrome takes to develop, the link between fatigue and polio may not be immediately apparent.

- Exercise designed to strengthen muscles can increase muscle strength in the postpolio syndrome patient. Energy conservation strategies designed to simplify activities of daily living may also be helpful.

- The dopamine agonist bromocriptine and the antiviral amantadine have both been studied in postpolio syndrome fatigue. Bromocriptine appears to reduce fatigue both on self-report

(continued)

Postpolio Syndrome: Key Concepts—Cont'd

measures and measures of cognitive functioning. Amantadine has also been shown to be beneficial in some patients, although the overall results of the study did not show a statistically significant effect.

---

a 6-week, double-blind trial of amantadine in 23 patients. Overall, 54% of those given amantadine versus 43% of those given placebo reported a decrease in fatigue; the difference was not significant.[18] Nevertheless, several patients in the amantadine group elected to continue therapy.

CONCLUSIONS

Fatigue, along with new onset muscle weakness, sensitivity to cold, and pain, are symptomatic of postpolio syndrome. The fatigue of postpolio syndrome appears most likely to be a late manifestation of the peripheral muscle damage caused by acute poliovirus infection. It can take years, or even decades, to manifest. Although more research needs to be performed on treatment, there is evidence that exercise, energy conservation strategies, and dopaminergic medications may be of some use for reducing fatigue.

REFERENCES

1. Clark K, Dinsmore G, Gramfan J, Dalakas MC. A personality profile of patients diagnosed with post-polio syndrome. Neurology 44:1809–1811, 1994.
2. Trojan DA, Cashman NR, Shapiro S, et al. Predictive factors for post-poliomyelitis syndrome. Arch Phys Med Rehabil 75:770–777, 1994.
3. Jubelt B, Drucker J. Post-polio syndrome: an update. Semin Neurol 13:283–290, 1993.
4. Ramlow J, Alexander M, LaPorte R, et al. Epidemiology of the post-polio syndrome. Am J Epidemiol 136:769–786, 1992.
5. Wekre LL, Stanghelle JK, Lobben B, Oyhaugen S. The Norwegian Polio Study 1994: a nationwide survey of problems in long-standing poliomyelitis. Spinal Cord 36:280–284, 1998.
6. Bruno RL, Frick NM, Cohen J. Polioencephalitis, stress, and the etiology of post-polio sequelae. Orthopedics 14:1269–1276, 1991.
7. Bruno RL. Abnormal movements in sleep as a post-polio sequelae. Am J Phys Med Rehabil 77:339–343, 1998.
8. Bruno RL, Galski T, DeLuca J. The neuropsychology of post-polio fatigue. Arch Phys Med Rehabil 74:1061–1065, 1993.
9. Sunnerhagen KS, Grimby G. Muscular effects in late polio. Acta Physiol Scand 171:335–340, 2001.
10. Bruno RL, Creange SJ, Frick NM. Parallels between post-polio fatigue and chronic fatigue syndrome: a common pathophysiology? Am J Med 105A:66S–73S, 1998.

11. Schanke AK. Psychological distress, social support and coping behavior among polio survivors: a 5-year perspective on 63 polio patients. Disabil Rehabil 19:108–116, 1997.

12. Bruno RL. Paralytic vs nonparalytic polio: distinction without a difference? Am J Phys Med Rehabil 79:4–12, 2000.

13. Packer TL, Martins I, Krefting L, Brouwer B. Activity and post-polio fatigue. Orthopedics 14:1223–1226, 1991.

14. Bartfeld H, Ma D. Recognizing postpolio syndrome. Hosp Practice (Off Ed) 31:95–97, 1996.

15. Milner-Brown HS. Muscle strengthening in a post-polio subject through a high-resistance weight-training program. Arch Phys Med Rehabil 74:1165–1167, 1993.

16. Halbritter T. Management of a patient with post-polio syndrome. J Am Acad Nurse Pract 13:555–559, 2001.

17. Bruno RL, Zimmerman JR, Creange SJ, et al. Bromocriptine in the treatment of post-polio fatigue: a pilot study with implications for the pathophysiology of fatigue. Am J Phys Med Rehabil 75:340–347, 1996.

18. Stein DP, Dambrosia JM, Dalakas MC. A double-blind, controlled trial of amantadine for the treatment of fatigue in patients with the post-polio syndrome. Ann NY Acad Sci 25:296–302, 1995.

Parkinson's Disease

Fatigue is a major symptom of Parkinson's disease (PD), occurring in two thirds of patients, with the majority of those with fatigue calling it the most disabling symptom of their disease.[1] Unfortunately, it is neither well understood nor well recognized by the treating physician. Data have shown that treating neurologists diagnosed fatigue accurately in only one quarter of fatigued patients during routine office visits.[2]

Fatigue and other nonmotor symptoms (i.e., anxiety, depression, sleep disorders, or sensory disturbances) are all common in PD patients. In fact, only a minority—approximately 10%—have been shown to have no nonmotor symptoms of the disease.[3] Although the cause remains poorly understood, fatigue appears to be a long-term phenomenon. In a 9-year follow-up of PD patients originally diagnosed with fatigue, the symptoms remained a persistent problem.[4] Fatigue does not appear to correlate with the severity or duration of PD, but as in other diseases, there is a moderate correlation with depression.[2]

As in multiple sclerosis (MS), it is possible the fatigue can have both peripheral and central components. There is evidence that PD–related fatigue is a central phenomenon, related to the central dopaminergic deficiencies of the disease.[1] Other researchers have hypothesized that it is a peripheral phenomenon related to mitochondrial dysfunction in the muscle.[5] Parkinson's symptoms such as muscle stiffness, tremor, and difficulty transferring can lead to individual muscle fatigue. Therefore, fatigue in PD should be considered multifactorial, with a primary form related to the loss of dopaminergic neurons in the substantia nigra, and the existence of secondary contributors such as excessive daytime sleepiness, medication use, deconditioning, the effort required in performing tasks of daily living, and simply the effects of older age, as PD onset does not generally occur in patients until their 50s.

Muscle disuse and deconditioning are challenges in the management of any PD patient. Underuse of muscles can lead to decrements in strength and stamina, and even atrophy, contributing to fatigue, which can in turn cause even greater deconditioning in a vicious cycle. It has been demonstrated that PD patients with more severe fatigue are more sedentary and have poorer functional capacity and physical function compared with patients with less fatigue [Garber CE, unpublished data].

Sleep disturbances are very common in PD patients, and can contribute significantly to feelings of fatigue. Excessive daytime sleepiness occurs in approximately 15% of PD patients.[6] In addition, PD patients may have trouble sleeping due to an inability to move comfortably during sleep (e.g., to roll over), and bladder dysfunction or tremor can interfere with the normal sleep cycle. Restless legs syndrome and periodic limb movements of sleep are also frequent in PD, as is REM sleep behavior disorder, which is characterized by sleep talking, shouting, and intense, sometimes violent movements.[7] It has been observed that patients with fatigue that is secondary to a sleep disorder generally feel most fatigued in the early afternoon, whereas those with fatigue unrelated to a sleep disorder do not experience variability in fatigue severity throughout the day [Garber CE, unpublished data].

A number of medications can cause feelings of fatigue and tiredness in PD. Dopaminergic medications, especially the dopamine agonists (e.g., pramipexole, ropinirole, bromocriptine), are significantly associated with somnolence.[8] Muscle relaxants such as benzodiazepines may cause tiredness. Fatigue may also appear near the end of a medication cycle; that is, when a patient is weaning off levodopa.

MANAGEMENT

There is little literature on management of the underlying primary fatigue disorder in PD. Effective management of associated factors such as sleep disturbances, motor symptoms, and depression can be helpful in reducing feelings of fatigue. Because of the high risk of sleep disturbances in PD, interviewing the patient's bed partner can be especially fruitful in uncovering a sleep disorder.

Dopaminergic medications have been shown to reduce the incidence of restless legs syndrome, although because they may increase the risk of somnolence, the physician should prescribe the lowest effective dose. Although the wake-promoting agent modafinil has not been tested specifically for Parkinson's-related fatigue, it has been shown to reduce excessive daytime sleepiness, a related disorder that has a high degree of overlap with fatigue.[9] Because modafinil promotes wakefulness, it may also allow physicians to increase the dose of dopaminergic medications, thereby reducing motor symptoms that interfere with sleep but carry a high risk of excessive daytime somnolence.[9] A trial of antidepressant medications can be used to treat associated depression, although it does not appear that fatigue itself generally responds to antidepressant therapy.[4]

A number of nonpharmacologic interventions may be of help (Table 9-1).[10] An exercise program should be instituted if possible, although patients may have trouble exercising due to motor symptoms such as tremor or freezing, and a general slowing of response. More difficult tasks can be performed when movements are likely to require less energy (i.e., following levodopa dosing or during an "on" period).

Table 9-1. Strategies that May Help Reduce Fatigue

Eat healthy to maintain energy

Participate in an exercise program that combines aerobic activity and stretching to the extent possible

Establish a regular bedtime; avoid frequent napping or stimulation at bedtime

Decrease caffeine and alcohol intake

Keep mentally active (boredom often leads to fatigue)

Seek assistance with tasks when necessary; do not force too many tasks into one time period

(Source: APDA Young Parkinson's Newsletters. Available on the Internet at http://members.aol.com/apdaypd/young/fatigue.htm. Last accessed July 23, 2002.)

Fatigue in Parkinson's Disease: Key Concepts

- Fatigue and other nonmotor symptoms of Parkinson's disease (PD) are experienced by 90% of PD patients. Fatigue appears to be a long-term symptom of PD that does not correlate well with the severity or duration of disease.
- Fatigue in PD may be a central phenomenon related to the loss of dopaminergic neurons in the substantia nigra, or a peripheral phenomenon related to mitochondrial dysfunction.
- Sleep disturbance is one of the most important contributors to fatigue in the PD patient. Factors that may interfere with sleep include tremor and movement disorders such as restless legs syndrome.
- Dopaminergic medications used to treat PD (e.g., dopamine agonists such as pramipexole) can cause excessive somnolence; it is important to reduce these medications to the lowest possible dose that effectively controls motor symptoms.
- Treatment options for PD include exercise therapy and energy-effectiveness strategies, as well as drugs such as modafinil, which can control excessive somnolence.

CONCLUSIONS

The large majority of PD patients experience non-motor symptoms of the disease, including fatigue. As in other disorders, fatigue in PD is related to a multitude of factors, including insults to the central nervous system caused by the disease itself, and secondary factors such as sleep disorders and deconditioning. The management program should be designed to carefully tailor the dosing of sedating dopaminergic medications, treat motor disturbances that can cause tiredness and pain, and address any psychological contributors.

REFERENCES

1. Ziv I, Avraham M, Michaelov Y, et al. Enhanced fatigue during motor performance in patients with Parkinson's disease. Neurology 51:1583–1586, 1998.
2. Shulman LM, Taback RL, Rabinstein AA, Weiner WJ. Nonrecognition of depression and other non-motor symptoms in Parkinson's disease. Parkinsonism Relat Disord 8:193–197, 2002.
3. Shulman LM, Taback RL, Bean J, Weiner WJ. Comorbidity of the nonmotor symptoms of Parkinson's disease. Mov Disord 16:507–510, 2001.
4. Friedman JH, Friedman H. Fatigue in Parkinson's disease: a nine-year follow-up. Mov Disord 16:1120–1122, 2001.
5. Schapira AH. Evidence for mitochondrial dysfunction in Parkinson's disease: a critical appraisal. Mov Disord 9:125–138, 1994.
6. Tandberg E, Larsen JP, Karlsen K. Excessive daytime sleepiness and sleep benefit in Parkinson's disease: a community-based study. Mov Disord 14:922–927, 1999.

7. Trendwalker C. Sleep dysfunction in Parkinson's disease. Clin Neurosci 5:107–114, 1998.
8. Schafer D, Greulich W. Effects of Parkinsonian medication on sleep. J Neurol 247(suppl 4):24–27, 2000.
9. Nieves AV, Lange AE. Treatment of excessive daytime sleepiness in patients with Parkinson's disease with modafinil. Clin Neuropharmacol 25(2):111–114, 2002.
10. APDA Young Parkinson's Newsletters. Available on the Internet at http://members.aol.com/apdaypd/young/fatigue.htm. Last accessed July 23, 2002.

Cancer-Related Fatigue

Fatigue has been called "the most important untreated symptom in cancer today."[1] Although improvements have been seen in a number of areas of cancer management, such as pain, depression, and nausea and vomiting, fatigue remains inadequately discussed and undertreated.[1] The reasons for this are varied. First, as with fatigue in most diseases, cancer-related fatigue is largely a subjective experience, and relies on self-reporting. Also, physicians and patients alike may view cancer-related fatigue as something to be endured, rather than a true symptom that requires an intervention. Third, it may be too easy to overlook a symptom such as fatigue when focusing on aggressive management of the tumor to ensure the patient's survival.

Physicians and patients both put the incidence of cancer-related fatigue at approximately 75% to 80% (Fig. 10-1).[2,3] However, they differ in the importance that they ascribe to fatigue. In one study, almost two thirds of patients reported that

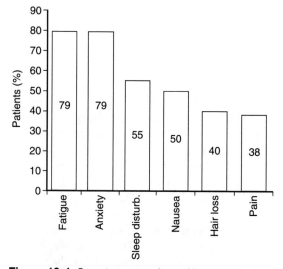

Figure 10-1. Symptoms experienced by cancer patients. (Reprinted with permission from Sobrero A, Puglisi F, Guglielmi A, et al. Fatigue: a main component of anemia symptomatology. Semin Oncol 28[suppl 8]: 15–18, 2001.)

fatigue affected their life more than pain; however, only 37% of the physicians believed this to be the case.[4] Fatigue also affects quality of life in the cancer patient more than nausea or depression.[2]

Attempts have been made to emphasize the vital importance of fatigue management in cancer patients, as studies have shown that patients do not simply experience fatigue, they *suffer* with it. The fatigue experienced by cancer patients can be very rapid in onset, intense in severity, and constitute an overwhelming energy drain, causing social, spiritual, psychological, and cognitive distress.[5]

Fatigue generally appears during the acute treatment period; however, it is not limited to this period, as approximately one third of cancer patients report chronic fatigue.[6] Interestingly, researchers have found that feelings of fatigue can *predate* a diagnosis of cancer,[7] suggesting that factors such as tumor growth may play a role in fatigue etiology.

CAUSES OF CANCER-RELATED FATIGUE

Guidelines on cancer-related fatigue from the National Comprehensive Cancer Network were published in 2000, and are also available on the

Internet at www.nccn.org.[8] Fatigue can be caused by a number of physical and psychological factors in the cancer patient (Table 10-1).[8] Psychologically, the depression and anxiety that may accompany a

Table 10-1. Causes of Fatigue in the Cancer Patient

Primary Factors
  Pain
  Emotional distress
  Anemia
  Sleep disturbance
  Hypothyroidism

Comorbidities
  Infection
  Cardiac dysfunction
  Pulmonary dysfunction
  Renal dysfunction
  Hepatic dysfunction
  Endocrine dysfunction

Nutritional/Metabolic Causes
  Changes in caloric intake/weight
  Fluid electrolyte imbalance (sodium, potassium, calcium, magnesium)

Conditioning Causes
  Changes in exercise or activity patterns
  Deconditioning

(Reprinted with permission from Atkinson A. NCCN Practice Guidelines for cancer-related fatigue. Oncology 14:151–161, 2000.)

diagnosis of cancer can cause fatigue. Anemia is a common side effect of both radiotherapy and chemotherapy, and is perhaps the most powerful physical contributor to fatigue. Anemia can also be caused by the absolute loss of iron-containing hemoglobin through surgery or phlebotomy for blood testing. The relationship between fatigue and anemia is so important that the majority of symptoms and signs on the anemia subscale of the Functional Assessment of Cancer Therapy Measurement System are related to fatigue (Table 10-2).[9]

Irrespective of anemia, both radiotherapy and chemotherapy can cause pain, loss of appetite, nausea, and malnutrition that weaken the patient, causing fatigue on their own or exacerbating fatigue stemming from other factors. Hormone therapy has also been associated with fatigue: In a study of 62 prostate cancer patients receiving cyproterone acetate and goserelin, mean fatigue scores on the Fatigue Severity Scale (FSS) increased significantly over the course of 3 months of therapy. Much of the fatigue could be attributed to an increase in psychological distress.[10]

Researchers have distinguished between self-reported mental fatigue (characterized by reduced motivation and mental exhaustion) and physical fatigue (characterized by increased limitations on activity). In one study of Swedish cancer patients,

Table 10-2. Functional Assessment of Cancer Therapy Measurement System: Anemia Subscale

Fatigue Component
Fatigue
Weakness
Tiredness
Listlessness
Low energy
Trouble finishing tasks
Requires assistance
Too tired to eat
Social limitation
Frustration with fatigue
Need help with usual activities
Need to sleep during the day

Nonfatigue component
Trouble walking
Dizziness
Headaches
Dyspnea
Chest pain
Libido
Motivation

(Reprinted with permission from Cella D. Factors influencing quality of life in cancer patients: anemia and fatigue. Semin Oncol 3[suppl 7]:43–46, 1998.)

physical fatigue factors were more pronounced than mental fatigue factors.[11] An interesting finding of this study was that fatigue scores peaked at the end of treatment after full radiotherapy doses were delivered. This is in accordance with studies showing that the frequency of fatigue increases over the course of radiation therapy.[12]

Limitations placed on the patient such as reduced mobility can reduce conditioning and thus decrease the body's oxygen-carrying capacity. It must also be emphasized that cancer patients undergoing surgery are subject to the same type of postoperative fatigue that other surgical patients experience, caused by a nonspecific stress reaction (see Chapter 11 for a more complete discussion).

The impact of cancer-related fatigue can be considerable, both economically and in terms of family adjustment. In a study by Curt et al., 75% of patients and 40% of caregivers had changed their employment status because of the patient's fatigue.[1] Nursing research has shown that family roles shift subtly, with the family taking over responsibilities and activities that the patient cannot perform because of fatigue.[13]

MANAGEMENT

The awareness of cancer-related fatigue appears to be increasing among physicians. Unfortunately, management in many cases remains inadequate. In one survey, physicians responded to hearing about their patients' fatigue by doing nothing or by recommending only rest.[2]

The comprehensive treatment of fatigue is discussed in more detail in Chapter 17, but some basic principles can be summarized here. Assessment of cancer-related fatigue should include its duration, pattern and course, as well as any exacerbating or alleviating factors.[2] As with most diseases with a fatigue component, assessment of sleep hygiene is appropriate because many factors (e.g., the presence of bed sores in patients who are bedridden) may interfere with sleep. The physician should look closely for evidence of a mood disorder that presents with fatigue; antidepressant therapy may be beneficial in these patients.

Pain management may increase pain-free movement and thus allow the patient to remain more mobile and better conditioned. It may also relieve depression and anxiety symptoms, both of which correlate with fatigue. However, many analgesics and opiate medications can contribute to tiredness. If high doses of pain medications are necessary, use of the wake-promoting agent modafinil or a psychostimulant may help overcome drug-induced somnolence.

A number of specific scales have been designed to assess cancer-related fatigue, including the Fatigue Symptom Inventory, Cancer Fatigue Scale, and the

Piper Fatigue Scale. The Cancer Fatigue Scale consists of 58 items divided along three subscales (physical, affective, and cognitive),[14] whereas the Piper Fatigue scale consists of 22 numerically scaled items (0 to 10) that measure four dimensions of fatigue (behavioral/severity, affective meaning, sensory, and cognitive/mood). The findings are presented as the numeric sum of each individual scale, along with a total score.[7,15] Other scales, including the FSS, have also been used in cancer populations.[10]

Several options exist to treat anemia, including recombinant human erythropoietin, which drives the process of red blood cell production in the erythroid marrow and stimulates the body to release iron stores. Supplemental iron therapy can also be given. Studies specifically in chemotherapy populations have shown that exogenous erythropoietin significantly improves hemoglobin levels; secondary analyses showed quality of life improvements.[16] In a recent large-scale study of more than 3000 chemotherapy patients with nonmyeloid malignancies, exogenous erythropoietin in a dose of 40,000 to 60,000 U once weekly significantly reduced fatigue as measured by the anemia subscale of the Functional Assessment of Cancer Therapy.[17]

Individual or group psychotherapy, relaxation therapy, and exercise all have some value in managing cancer-related fatigue, as does concomitant treatment of insomnia, dehydration, malnutrition, and infection.[8] Therefore, an appropriate multidisciplinary intervention involving the physician, nurse, and social worker may have an impact on reducing fatigue.[18]

Several studies have demonstrated the specific benefits of exercise in cancer patients. In one study of 72 breast cancer patients undergoing an exercise program, the intensity of fatigue declined significantly with increasing exercise endurance.[19] Exercise programs may even be appropriate for cancer patients with advanced disease. In one study of patients in a hospice program, a carefully tailored exercise program (e.g., consisting of walking 5 minutes, performing arm exercises in a chair, or marching on the spot) resulted in slight decreases in fatigue and improvements in activity over 28 days. There was also a potential trend toward reduced anxiety on the Hospital Anxiety and Depression Scale.[20]

CONCLUSION

Fatigue has a profound impact on functioning in the cancer patient, and is a symptom that must be addressed. Radiation and chemotherapy can both cause meylosuppression and subsequent anemia-related fatigue, and factors such as pain, loss of appetite, and psychological distress are significant contributing factors. A multidisciplinary program that provides exercise, proper nutrition, correction of anemia, and psychological interventions when appropriate can reduce fatigue and increase functioning in the cancer patient.

Cancer-Related Fatigue: Key Concepts

- It is easy to overlook the importance of fatigue in the cancer patient, given the threat to life caused by cancer itself. However, fatigue must be addressed, as it can be an overwhelming energy drain and has a major impact on quality of life.
- Fatigue in the cancer patient can be caused by the enormous energy required by the body to fight cancer. Other contributors are anemia (caused by radiation or chemotherapy), pain, sleep disturbances, emotional distress, depression, hypothyroidism, reduced calorie intake, deconditioning, and endocrine dysfunction.
- Reducing fatigue in the cancer patient requires a multidisciplinary approach that involves proper and adequate nutrition, correction of anemia, pain management, exercise, and counseling. The physician, nurse, social worker, nutritionist, and physical therapist all should play a role in fatigue management.

REFERENCES

1. Curt GA, Breitbart W, Cella D, et al. Impact of cancer-related fatigue on the lives of patients: new findings from the Fatigue Coalition. Oncologist 5:353–360, 2000.

2. Curt GA. Fatigue in cancer: like pain, this is a symptom that physicians can and should manage. BMJ 322:1560, 2001.

3. Sobrero A, Puglisi F, Guglielmi A, et al. Fatigue: a main component of anemia symptomatology. Semin Oncol 28(suppl 8):15–18, 2001.

4. Vogelzang NJ, Breitbart W, Cella D, et al. Patient, caregiver, and oncologist perceptions of cancer-related fatigue: results of a triparte assessment survey. Semin Hematol 34(suppl 2):4–12, 1997.

5. Holley S. Cancer-related fatigue: suffering a different fatigue. Cancer Pract 8:87–95, 2000.

6. Jereczek-Fossa BA, Marsiglia HR, Orecchia R. Radiotherapy-related fatigue: how to assess and how to treat the symptom: a commentary. Tumori 87:147–151, 2001.

7. Piper BG, Lindsey AM, Dodd MJ, et al. The development of an instrument to measure the subjective dimension of fatigue. In Funk SG, Tourquist EM, Champagne M, et al. (eds.). Key Aspects of Comfort: Management of Pain and Nausea. New York: Springer, 1989, pp 199–208.

8. Atkinson A. NCCN Practice Guidelines for cancer-related fatigue. Oncology 14:151–161, 2000.

9. Cella D. Factors influencing quality of life in cancer patients: anemia and fatigue. Semin Oncol 3 (suppl 7):43–46, 1998.

10. Stone P, Hardy J, Huddart R, et al. Fatigue in patients with prostate cancer receiving hormone therapy. Eur J Cancer 36:1134–1141, 2000.

11. Furst CJ, Ashberg E. Dimensions of fatigue during radiotherapy: an application of the multidimensional Fatigue Inventory. Support Care Cancer 9:355–360, 2001.

12. King KG, Nail LM, Kreamer K, et al. Patients' descriptions of the experience of receiving radiation therapy. Oncol Nurs Forum 12: 55–61, 1985.

13. Hamilton J, Butler L, Wagenaar H, et al. The impact of cancer-related fatigue on patients and their families. Can Oncol Nurs J 11:192–198, 2001.

14. Okuyama T, Akechi T, Kugaya A, et al. Factors correlated with fatigue in disease-free breast cancer patients: application of the Cancer Fatigue Scale. Support Care Cancer 8:215–222, 2000.

15. Monga U, Kerrigan AJ, Thornby J, Monga TN. Prospective study of fatigue in localized prostate cancer patients undergoing radiotherapy. Radiation Oncol Invest 7:178–185, 1999.

16. Abels R. Erythropoietin for anemia in cancer patients: Eur J Cancer 29(suppl 2):1616–1634, 1993.

17. Gabrilove JL, Cleeland CS, Livingston RB, et al. Clinical evaluation of once-weekly dosing of epoetin alfa in chemotherapy patients: improvements in hemoglobin and quality of life are similar to three-times-weekly dosing. J Clin Oncol 19:2875–2882, 2001.

18. Grant M, Golant M, Rivera L, et al. Developing a community program on cancer pain and fatigue. Cancer Pract 8:187–194, 2000.

19. Schwartz AL, Mori M, Gao R, et al. Exercise reduces daily fatigue in women with breast cancer receiving chemotherapy. Med Sci Sports Exerc 33:718–723, 2001.
20. Porock D, Kristjanson LJ, Tinnelly K, et al. An exercise intervention for advanced cancer patients experiencing fatigue: a pilot study. J Palliative Care 16:30–36, 2000.

CHAPTER ELEVEN

Postoperative Fatigue

Fatigue is a common occurrence after surgery. Although this is an almost intuitive statement, given the physical trauma and psychological stress of surgery, fatigue is often overlooked in the face of more tangible symptoms such as pain. According to some surveys, up to three fourths of patients experience moderate-to-severe fatigue in the weeks after surgery, yet it is often simply not addressed.[1] For example, in a study of patients recovering from hysterectomy, postoperative fatigue was discussed with only about two thirds of the individuals, and more than half of the patients were not offered any treatments or recommendations to alleviate their fatigue.[1]

The fatigue of the postoperative period is associated with the now familiar covariates, including pain, anxiety, fear, depression, and activity limita-tions.[2] If present before surgery, fatigue can have a powerful influence on recovery (Fig. 11-1). For example, higher degrees of preoperative fatigue, combined with greater anxiety and poorer preoper-ative function, were shown to lead to a longer recovery time after hip arthroplasty.[3] Fatigue, along with pain, can delay the return to work even after laparoscopic procedures.[4]

Sleep loss is an additional contributing factor: In another sample of 38 men undergoing coronary artery bypass grafting who were experiencing sleep

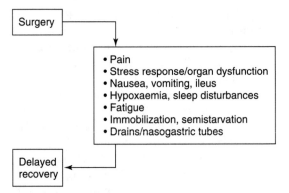

Figure 11-1. Fatigue is a significant contributor to postoperative morbidity. (Reprinted with permission from Willmore DW. Management of patients in fast track surgery. BMJ 322:473–476, 2001.)

loss, 80% had at least moderate anxiety before surgery and approximately 15% were depressed. Those who were anxiety prone continued to exhibit anxious reactivity after surgery, and had symptoms of cognitive and behavioral fatigue, as well as sleep problems. (Significantly, the presence of postoperative cognitive/behavioral fatigue was predictive of a higher New York Heart Association [NYHA] class.)[5]

The psychological contributors to postoperative fatigue are undeniably significant. However, most research in this area has focused on the myriad physiologic reasons for fatigue. The emergence of postoperative fatigue appears to be related in large part to a nonspecific reaction brought on by the body's physiologic response to stress. Postoperative evaluations of patients undergoing major surgery have shown marked increases in plasma free tryptophan, a serotonin precursor that is involved in fatigue and sleep.[6] Elevated levels of the proinflammatory cytokine interleukin-6 were also seen following laparoscopically assisted vaginal and abdominal hysterectomy.[7] In another study of those who underwent coronary artery bypass surgery, postoperative fatigue was predicted by high preoperative levels of noradrenaline.[8]

The muscle weakness caused by postoperative disuse can increase muscle fatigue following exertion. Fatigue after surgery can accompany a fall in nutrition status, with these patients losing more weight and skinfold thickness. This can not only induce weakness from caloric deficiency, but can cause catabolic changes through neuroendocrine mechanisms.[8] Poor nutrition in the postoperative period can contribute to weakness and prolonged recovery, and lack of mobility during the recovery period leads to deconditioning and less efficient oxygen use. Loss of blood during and after the procedure can also cause anemia-related fatigue.

Adjuvant preoperative and postoperative therapies are also major causes of fatigue in the surgical patient. Although the fatigue of cancer-related therapies is discussed in more depth in Chapter 10, it is worth mentioning here that fatigue and lethargy are complications of preoperative radiation therapy, as well as postoperative adjuvant therapy.[9] Preoperative radiation therapy exhibits a detrimental effect on work capacity and physical performance,[10] most likely through anemia-related mechanisms.

Although fatigue can be an issue with any form of surgery, it has been demonstrated most often in gynecologic and cardiac surgery. Clinical studies and patient surveys have shown that fatigue, diminished energy levels, an increased need for rest, and difficulty performing daily routines are prevalent after gynecologic surgery and persist for weeks to months. Persistent and debilitating fatigue in the early preoperative period following hysterectomy is even more common than pain,[11] and has been shown to interfere with daily activities, and to increase feelings of frustration, depression, and difficulty concentrating.[1]

Cardiac surgery, even when considered successful in improving overall health status, has been shown to cause fatigue and persistent sleep disturbances in older patients.[12] Fatigue may be related to actual changes in heart function after cardiac surgery, with increased levels of fatigue correlating with increases in heart rate for a given amount of work, possibly related to the nonspecific effects of deconditioning.[8]

MANAGEMENT

Unlike the primary fatigue of other disorders such as multiple sclerosis, the fatigue of the postoperative period is normally limited in duration, and should be expected to improve with time. Symptoms are generally worst in the first postoperative week. However, a substantial percentage of patients do experience fatigue for many months.[8]

The potential treatment options for postoperative fatigue should address the underlying causes, and include a return to activity and a plan to improve conditioning as soon as practicable after the procedure (Box 11-1). Early and adequate nutrition is also important. If blood laboratory tests indicate anemia, the patient can be treated with oral iron supplements (although these may produce

---

Box 11-1. Strategies to Manage Fatigue in the Postoperative Patient

1. **Educate the patient:** The patient should be educated about the causes of fatigue in the postoperative period (e.g., anemia, pain, depression, prolonged stress). The patient should be reassured that fatigue is a normal part of the postoperative period and is self-limiting in almost all cases.

2. **Use minimally invasive techniques:** Whenever possible, the surgeon and anesthesiologist should employ minimally invasive techniques (e.g., laparoscopy versus laparotomy, epidural or local anesthesia versus general anesthesia). These techniques reduce recovery time, minimize the body's stress response, and allow a faster return to normal activity.

3. **Treat anemia:** Anemia caused by blood loss during surgery and blood drawing for preoperative testing is a major physical contributor to postoperative fatigue. Anemia can be treated with iron supplements, exogenous erythropoietin, and folic acid (see Chapter 17 for more details on recommended doses).

(continued)

Box 11-1. Strategies to Manage Fatigue in the Postoperative Patient—Cont'd

---

4. **Ensure an adequate diet:** A nutrition program that ensures adequate calories can help maintain strength during the recovery period. For patients who have lost their appetite, an appetite stimulant (such as a selective serotonin reuptake inhibitor) may be tried.

5. **Consider perioperative steroid use:** Data have shown that perioperative use of intravenous methylprednisolone (60 to 90 minutes before the operation) can reduce the body's stress response and thereby reduce postoperative fatigue.

6. **Get the patient moving:** Early postoperative mobilization can help reduce fatigue resulting from muscle disuse and help patients maintain their strength. If ambulation is not possible, physical therapy consisting of range-of-motion exercises may be performed in bed with the aid of a physical therapist.

7. **Control contributors to fatigue:** These include postoperative pain, depression, and sleep difficulties. Adequate analgesia should be maintained at all times, and antidepressant therapy can be used if the patient shows signs of depression (or anxiety). Medications to aid sleep can be prescribed, making sure to choose agents that do not interfere with muscle strength or balance.

gastrointestinal side effects), vitamin B_{12}, or exogenous erythropoietin, which has been shown to correct anemia after major gynecologic surgery.[13]

Data have suggested that high-dose intravenous methylprednisolone in the perioperative period (60 to 90 minutes before operation) can reduce the body's stress response after abdominal surgery. Fatigue in those receiving high-dose steroids was reduced by half in the first day after the operation, and marked reductions were seen in markers of the stress response, including C-reactive protein and T-cell activation.[14]

There has been much recent interest in developing comprehensive multidisciplinary strategies to facilitate surgical recovery. "Fast track" surgery aims to reduce or avoid fatigue and other sequelae of the stress response and organ dysfunction, thereby shortening the time for a full recovery and avoiding fatigue. Techniques involve the use of epidural or regional anesthesia instead of general anesthesia, use of minimally invasive techniques, optimal pain control, and aggressive postoperative rehabilitation, including early oral nutrition and ambulation.[15]

Such strategies have been successful in managing contributors to fatigue. In a study of 14 patients who underwent colonic resection with an accelerated recovery program and 14 patients who received conventional care, those who underwent the accelerated program had a smaller reduction in lean body mass, pulmonary function, and oxygenation, and retained their level of exercise performance. In contrast, exercise performance decreased by nearly half in the conventional recovery group.[16]

Nevertheless, less invasive means of surgery are not necessarily a predictor of lower fatigue in the postoperative period. In a study of 35 individuals who were assigned to coronary artery bypass grafting or minimally invasive direct coronary artery bypass, both groups reported fatigue, shortness of breath, and pain as major symptoms postdischarge.[17]

CONCLUSION

Fatigue in the postoperative patient is a common occurrence that is often inadequately addressed by the surgeon and postoperative care team. Although anemia resulting from blood loss is a major physical cause, pain, a sustained stress response, and activity limitations also contribute to fatigue. A specific management plan should be devised that educates the patient and family on fatigue during the postoperative period, encourages early mobilization, and addresses contributing factors such as postoperative pain.

REFERENCES

1. DeCherney AH, Bachmann G, Isaacson K, Gall S. Postoperative fatigue negatively impacts the daily lives of patients recovering from hysterectomy. Obstet Gynecol 99:51–57, 2002.

2. Salmon P, Hall GM. Postoperative fatigue is a component of the emotional response to surgery: results of multivariate analysis. J Psychosom Res 50:325–335, 2001.

3. Salmon P, Hall GM, Peerbhoy D. Influence of the emotional response to surgery on functional recovery during 6 months after hip arthroplasty. J Behav Med 24:489–502, 2001.

4. Bisgaard T, Klarskov B, Rosenberg J, Kehlet H. Factors determining convalescence after uncomplicated laparoscopic cholecystectomy. Arch Surg 136: 917–921, 2001.

5. Edell-Gustafsson UM, Hetta JE. Anxiety, depression and sleep in male patients undergoing coronary artery bypass surgery. Scand J Caring Sci 13: 137–143, 1999.

6. Castell LM, Yamamoto T, Phoenix J, Newsholme EA. The role of tryptophan in fatigue in different conditions of stress. Adv Exp Med Biol 467: 697–704, 1999.

7. Rorarius MG, Kujansuu E, Baer GA, et al. Laparoscopically assisted vaginal and abdominal hysterectomy: comparison of postoperative pain, fatigue, and systemic response: a case-control study. Eur J Anaesthesiol 18:530–539, 2001.

8. Wessely S, Hotopf M, Sharpe M. Chronic Fatigue and its Syndromes. London: Oxford University Press, 1999.

9. Ooi BS, Tjandra JJ, Green MD. Morbidities of adjuvant chemotherapy and radiotherapy for resectable rectal cancer: an overview. Dis Colon Rectum 42:403–418, 1999.

10. Liedman B, Johnsson E, Merke C, et al. Preoperative adjuvant radiochemotherapy may increase the risk in patients undergoing thoracoabdominal esophageal resections. Dig Surg 18:169–175, 2001.

11. Rock JA. Quality-of-life assessment in gynecologic surgery. J Reprod Med 46(5 suppl):515–519, 2001.

12. Chocron S, Tatou E, Schjoth B, et al. Perceived health status in patients over 70 before and after open-heart operations. Age Ageing 29:329–334, 2000.

13. Stovall TG. Clinical experience with epoetin alfa in the management of hemoglobin levels in orthopedic surgery and cancer: implications for use in gynecologic surgery. J Reprod Med 46 (suppl 5):531–538, 2001.

14. Nagelschmidt M, Fu ZX, Saad S, et al. Preoperative high dose methylprednisolone improves patients outcomes after abdominal surgery. Eur J Surg 165:971–978, 1999.

15. Willmore DW, Kehlert H. Management of patients in fast track surgery. BMJ 322:473–476, 2001.

16. Basse L, Raskov HH, Jakobsen D, et al. Accelerated postoperative recovery programme after colonic resection improves physical performance, pulmonary function and body composition. Br J Surg 89:446–453, 2002.

17. Zimmerman L, Barnason S, Brey BA, et al. Comparison of recovery patterns for patients undergoing coronary artery bypass grafting and minimally invasive direct coronary artery bypass in the early discharge period. Prog Cardiovasc Nurs 17:132–141, 2002.

Systemic Lupus Erythematosus

Systemic lupus erythematosus (SLE) is a chronic autoimmune and rheumatic disorder characterized by unpredictable symptoms, including the characteristic "butterfly rash," joint pain and swelling, kidney and liver malfunctioning, hypertension, and impaired cerebral blood flow.[1] Despite this array of physical signs and symptoms, fatigue is often the presenting complaint. The incidence of fatigue in SLE rivals that for multiple sclerosis (MS), and as in MS, it is one of the most disabling symptoms. Up to 80% of SLE patients have reported fatigue.[2]

CAUSES OF FATIGUE IN SLE

The cause of fatigue in SLE is not known, but as in most diseases, it probably is caused by a complex mix of factors. The link between fatigue and the pathophysiologic processes of SLE is not clear; some physicians have reported that fatigue increases during a disease flare up,[1] or is associated with increased disease activity.[3] Factors contributing to fatigue include mood disorders, the deconditioning that comes from the physical limitations of this chronic disease, and associated fibromyalgia.[2] An association has also been reported with smoking, pain, and use of medications such as psychotropic drugs,[4] as well as headache.[5]

Reports of poor sleep quality are often associated with fatigue in SLE. According to some series, two thirds of SLE patients report poor sleep, which correlates at least moderately with fatigue scores.[2] Sleep disruption in SLE can result from muscle and joint pain, the presence of anxiety or depression, the use of corticosteroid therapy, and activity of the autonomic nervous system, causing breathlessness, sweating, and heart palpitations.[2,6]

Affective disorders can have a significant effect on fatigue, and they are recognized as prevalent problems in SLE by the American College of Rheumatology.[7] Mood disorders may be a neuropsychiatric manifestation of SLE related to the disease process itself, or the result of stresses arising from having a chronic illness. It has been suggested that it is the presence of depression, and not the presence of SLE per se, that is the determining factor for fatigue.[8]

Fatigue is by no means a benign symptom of SLE: Studies strongly point to a correlation between increasing fatigue and decreasing physical and mental functioning.[4] Fatigue can also be a result of the difficulties experienced by patients adjusting to chronic disease. In a study by Zonana-Nacach and colleagues, fatigue was associated with abnormal illness-related behaviors such as denial and affective disturbance, as well as learned helplessness.[4] These difficulties in adjustment are likely to contribute to the emergence of fatigue, and sustain established symptoms (Fig. 12-1).[4]

Quality of life is also clearly affected by fatigue, although it is not clear whether quality of life reductions are a cause or a result of fatigue. Deconditioning plays a significant role, and it has been reported that SLE patients have aerobic fitness levels approximately 65% of normal capacity.

The associations among SLE, fatigue, and fibromyalgia are intriguing but not well understood. Signs and symptoms of fibromyalgia are reported in approximately one fourth of SLE patients, and fibromyalgia, when it occurs with SLE, probably contributes to fatigue. In fact, it has been suggested that, as with depression, fibromyalgia provides the necessary "link" between SLE and fatigue symptoms.[8]

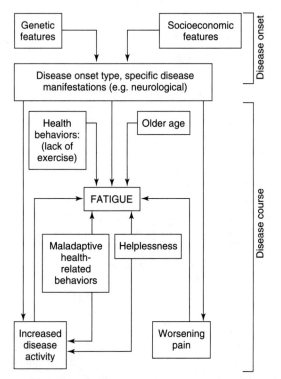

Figure 12-1. An explanatory model of fatigue and its relationship with disease activity. Factors such as learned helplessness and maladaptive health-related behaviors are likely to sustain fatigue symptoms over the course of systemic lupus erythematosus (SLE). (Reprinted with permission from Zonana-Nacach A, Roseman JM, McGwin G, et al. Systemic lupus erythematosus in three ethnic groups, VI: factors associated with fatigue within 5 years of criteria diagnosis. Lupus 9:101–109, 2000.)

The level of fatigue in SLE can be very severe. In one study, the mean fatigue score on the Fatigue Severity Scale (FSS) was 5.3 (generally, a score of ≥4 suggests the presence of severe fatigue).[4] Although the incidence of fatigue is similar among ethnic groups, the perceived severity may differ, with Caucasians reporting higher mean FSS scores than Hispanic or African-American patients (Fig. 12-2).[4]

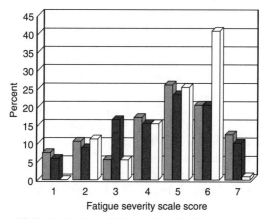

Figure 12-2. Distribution of Fatigue Severity Scale scores among Hispanic (*in grey*), African-American (*in black*), and Caucasian (*in white*) patients in the Lupus in Minority Population: Nature versus Nurture (LUMINA) cohort. (Reprinted with permission from Zonana-Nacach A, Roseman JM, McGwin G, et al. Systemic lupus erythematosus in three ethnic groups, VI: factors associated with fatigue within 5 years of criteria diagnosis. Lupus 9:101–109, 2000.)

RELATIONSHIP WITH DISEASE ACTIVITY

Whether fatigue increases with increasing disease activity in SLE remains an open question, with studies on the subject producing varying results. Some researchers have suggested that proinflammatory cytokines such as interleukin-1, which are activated by the autoimmune processes of SLE, promote sleep and fatigue. Therefore, increases in these disease markers may lead to increases in fatigue.[9] However, a study using the FSS as a measure of fatigue failed to find a significant association between fatigue and laboratory measures of disease activity (although fatigue did correlate with physicians' rating of disease activity).[3] Others have failed to find a correlation using measures of SLE activity including the SLE Disease Activity Index (SLEDAI)[8] and the Systemic Lupus Activity Measure (SLAM).

Nevertheless, some authors have concluded that a relationship between disease activity and fatigue severity does exist.[1] Overall, conclusions in this area are complicated by the fact that commonly used measures of SLE disease activity, such as the SLAM, themselves incorporate fatigue as a component of the disease assessment. Because the link between disease activity and fatigue is not clear, and because patients with quiescent SLE do experience fatigue,[2] the severity or duration of SLE should not be used as a fatigue predictor. Instead, the physician should always be attuned to the potential presence of fatigue, and assess the patient for this symptom regardless of the disease stage.

MANAGEMENT CONSIDERATIONS

The treatment of SLE itself involves a mixture of antimalarials and low-dose corticosteroids to keep disease activity at a minimum; immunosuppressives are used when multisystem involvement is seen.[2] Because fatigue (as well as depression) in SLE may represent the co-occurrence of fibromyalgia, it is worthwhile to conduct a fibromyalgia workup, assessing the patient for musculoskeletal pain and the presence of tender joints by manual examination.[4] In addition, the physician should be alert to the possibility of hypothyroidism and treatable causes of anemia, both of which, like SLE, are more common in women and may go undiagnosed.[2] Evaluations for comorbid mood or sleep disorders can help identify potential causes of fatigue.[10]

Unfortunately, little research has been performed on the treatment of fatigue in the SLE patient. The general treatment guidelines for fatigue that are discussed in Chapter 17 of this book are an excellent place to start in terms of a management

Fatigue and Systemic Lupus Erythematosus: Key Concepts

- Fatigue in the systemic lupus erythematosus (SLE) patient is likely caused by a complex mix of factors, including disease activity, mood and sleep disorders, physical deconditioning, and behaviors such as learned helplessness that the patient adopts as the result of chronic disease.
- The physician should assess poor sleep quality in the SLE patient as a potential cause of fatigue and treat the underlying disorder to attempt to alleviate fatigue. Sleep disruption can be caused by muscle and joint pain, affective disorders (depression and/or anxiety), or autonomic nervous system dysfunction.
- As in other diseases, affective disorders can have a significant effect on fatigue in the SLE patient. Proper identification and treatment of these disorders may reduce fatigue.
- Abnormal illness-related behaviors such as learned helplessness can contribute to fatigue and also sustain it. Referral for psychological testing and counseling/cognitive behavior therapy may help the patient recognize and work to change these behaviors.
- SLE patients may have poor aerobic fitness levels as a result of their disease, which can be a cause of fatigue. An exercise program that emphasizes improvements in aerobic capacity, flexibility, and muscle strength may help relieve fatigue.

program. A combination of an exercise program to increase energy reserves can prove effective, and strategies designed to alleviate depression or other mood symptoms are indicated when a mood disorder is suspected.

CONCLUSION

Fatigue is a prevalent symptom of SLE whose cause remains elusive. It likely stems from a complex interplay of physical deconditioning, sleep disorders, mood disorders, pain, disease activity, and behaviors such as learned helplessness that are adopted as a result of chronic disease. Although measures such as the FSS can help quantify the perceived severity of this symptom, the strategies for management are not well defined. Strategies that have been adopted for fatigue in other illness, including psychological therapy, exercise therapy, alleviation of mood symptoms, and wake-promoting/stimulant medications, may prove fruitful for symptom relief.

REFERENCES

1. Tayer WG, Nicassio PM, Weisman MH, et al. Disease status predicts fatigue in systemic lupus erythematosus. J Rheumatol 28:1999–2007, 2001.

2. Tench CM, McCurdie I, White PD, D'cruz DP. The prevalence and associations of fatigue in systemic lupus erythematosus. Rheumatology 39:1249–1254, 2000.

3. Krupp LB, LaRocca NG, Muir J, Steinberg AD. A study of fatigue in systemic lupus erythematosus. J Rheumatol 17:1450–1452, 1990.

4. Zonana-Nacach A, Roseman JM, McGwin G, et al. Systemic lupus erythematosus in three ethnic groups, VI: factors associated with fatigue within 5 years of criteria diagnosis. Lupus 9:101–109, 2000.

5. Amit M, Molad Y, Levy O, Wysenbeck AJ. Headache in systemic lupus erythematosus and its relation to other disease manifestations. Clin Exp Rheumatol 17:467–470, 1999.

6. Gudbjornsson B, Hetta J. Sleep disturbances in patients with systemic lupus erythematosus: a questionnaire-based study. Clin Exp Rheumatol 19:509–514, 2001.

7. American College of Rheumatology. Ad hoc committee. The American College of Rheumatology nomenclature and case definitions for neuropsychiatric lupus syndromes. Arthritis Rheum 42:599–608, 1999.

8. Wang B, Gladdman DD, Urowitz MG. Fatigue in lupus is not correlated with disease activity. J Rheumatol 25:892–895, 1998.

9. Wysenbeck AJ, Leibovici L, Weinberger A, Guedj D. Fatigue in systemic lupus erythematosus: prevalence and relation to disease expression. Br J Rheumatol 32:633–635, 1993.

10. McKinley P, Ouellette SC, Winkel G. The contributions of disease activity, sleep patterns and depression to fatigue in systemic lupus erythematosus. Arthritis Rheum 38: 826–834, 1995.

Lyme Disease

Infectious disorders are classic illnesses in which fatigue is prominent and probably accounts for most of the fatigue that occurs in otherwise healthy individuals. Examination of specific infectious disorders such as Lyme disease provides an opportunity to analyze the different ways the symptom may develop in the course of an illness.

Lyme disease is a multisystemic disorder caused by *Borrelia burgdorferi* that is spread primarily in the Northeastern United States by the deer tick *Ixodes scapularis.* Lyme disease is characterized by distinct phases: a localized acute infection, a disseminated later stage of infection, and a post-treatment chronic state. In the acute phase, Lyme disease is characterized by a flat, reddish rash (erythema migrans), which occurs at the site of the tick bite and typically spreads. The rash can develop 3 to 30 days after the tick bite and can be accompanied by generalized body symptoms such as fatigue, fever, muscle aches, and headache.

Fatigue also appears to be a common complication of the disease phase in which dissemination has occurred. Disseminated Lyme disease refers to the stage of infection when the organism has spread beyond the localized skin area where initial portal of entry occurred and involves the synovial fluid (joints), the nervous system, and the cardiac system. Patients with disseminated infection have higher rates of fatigue than patients with localized infection. Fatigue also tends to persist longer in patients in whom the diagnosis and treatment is delayed.

A more controversial and less well understood entity is post-Lyme syndrome (PLS), a condition characterized by severe fatigue, malaise, and cognitive complaints that follow Lyme disease cases and that persist 6 months or more after completion of antibiotic therapy.[1] In one series by Dattwyler and colleagues, 46 of 54 patients with late Lyme borreliosis complained of fatigue.[2] In a study that compared 38 patients who had Lyme disease for a mean duration of 6.2 years with 43 control patients, the Lyme disease patients had significantly more fatigue (26% vs 9%; $P = 0.04$), as well as more arthralgias and greater concentration difficulties.[3]

Other studies have reported even higher rates of fatigue in the PLS population. However, the area is not without controversy, as data have shown that the incidence of fatigue and other nonspecific symptoms (e.g., numbness, pain, muscle problems) may not actually be higher in those with PLS than in those in the general population. One of the largest and most comprehensive studies to date in PLS involved 678 patients with suspected Lyme disease of more than 4 years' duration. Symptoms including fatigue and pain that interfered with daily activities were reported by almost 70% of the participants. However, the researchers determined that only a minority of these (fewer than 20%) was attributable to Lyme disease.[4]

Outcomes like this lie at the heart of what is currently a great deal of controversy about long-term outcomes from Lyme disease. While some take the position that Lyme disease is a difficult-to-treat illness and can lead to a high degree of long-term complications such as fatigue, others have viewed Lyme disease as a much more treatable illness, and believe that patients with such long-term sequelae as fatigue either had been misdiagnosed with Lyme disease or that Lyme disease is not the cause of the symptom.[4]

This is supported, at least in part, by the fact that serologic tests for Lyme disease have a relatively low degree of specificity.[4] It is also supported by the fact that PLS has a high degree of overlap with other diseases of nonspecific symptomatology, such as chronic fatigue syndrome (CFS)[1] and fibromyalgia.[5] Both Lyme disease and CFS are heterogenous with respect to the severity of their clinical fatigue and other factors such as psychiatric disturbance and cognitive difficulties.[1] The data on antibiotic treatment unfortunately do not add significantly more clarity to this issue of whether PLS is a "real" disease or whether patients are exhibiting nonspecific symptoms of some other disease. Donta and colleagues found some degree of success with antibiotic use in treating fatigue and other chronic symptoms in PLS patients.[6,7] In this author's own research, we randomized 55 post-Lyme patients with severe fatigue to treatment with ceftriaxone or placebo. Patients randomized to the antibiotic did show improvement in their fatigue compared with placebo. However, a high number of adverse events were seen, causing 7% to be hospitalized from adverse effects. In addition, although the improvements in fatigue were encouraging, there were no improvements in impaired cognitive functioning or laboratory measures of infection, mitigating against the use of repeated antibiotic courses to address fatigue in this group.[8] Absent of any clinical signs of continuing infection, treatment of fatigue with continued courses of antibiotics is not supported by the literature.[9]

Fatigue in Lyme Disease: Key Concepts

- Fatigue and other generalized symptoms of infection can occur during the acute stages of Lyme disease (generally within 30 days of the deer tick bite).

- Fatigue is common in those with disseminated Lyme infection (when the organism has spread beyond the initial site of infection. Affected sites can include the joints, nervous system, and cardiac system).

- Fatigue lasts longer when treatment is delayed; therefore, a thorough skin examination along with a patient history should be performed in order to identify acute Lyme disease signs as quickly as possible and to initiate antibiotic therapy.

- Post-Lyme syndrome (PLS) is characterized by severe fatigue, malaise, and cognitive difficulties that persist at least 6 months after antibiotic treatment for the infection is completed. PLS is not well understood and its actual association with Lyme disease itself is controversial.

- Although the cause of PLS may be a mystery, it is important never to dismiss the patient's complaints. A thorough workup should be performed, paying close attention to those covariables (pain, sleep disorders, depression, and other psychological difficulties such as maladaptive coping skills).

- There is some evidence that antibiotic therapy in the PLS patient may improve fatigue. Overall, however, the literature does not support a role for continued courses of antibiotic therapy.

MANAGEMENT CONSIDERATIONS

Regardless of the source of fatigue in a patient who presents with PLS, the first tenet of fatigue management is to take seriously the patient's complaints of fatigue. Patients who present with PLS should be queried about the now-familiar contributors to fatigue, including pain, mood disorders, and sleep disorders, and if any of these are present, they should be treated appropriately. Psychotherapeutic approaches such as cognitive-behavioral therapy may be suggested, while a trial of a wake-promoting agent such as modafinil, although not tested in PLS, may be a reasonable course of action.

REFERENCES

1. Gaudino EA, Coyle PK, Krupp LB. Post-lyme syndrome and chronic fatigue syndrome: neuropsychiatric similarities and differences. Arch Neurol 54:1372–1376, 1997.
2. Dattwyler RJ, Volkman DJ, Halperin JJ, Luft BJ. Treatment of late Lyme borreliosis: a randomized comparison of ceftriaxone and penicillin. Lancet 1:1191–1194, 1988.
3. Shadick NA, Phillips CB, Logigian EL, et al. The long-term clinical outcomes of Lyme disease: a population-based retrospective cohort study. Ann Intern Med 121:560–567, 1994.

4. Seltzer EG, Gerber MA, Cartter ML, et al. Long-term outcomes of persons with Lyme disease. JAMA 283: 609–616, 2000.

5. Dinerman H, Steere AC. Lyme disease associated with fibromyalgia. Ann Intern Med 117:281–285, 1992.

6. Donta ST. Long-term outcomes of Lyme disease (Letter). JAMA 283:3068, 2000.

7. Donta ST. Tetracycline therapy of chronic Lyme disease. Clin Infect Dis 25(suppl 1):S52–S56, 1997.

8. Krupp LB. Presented at: the 54th Annual Meeting of the American Academy of Neurology, Denver, Colorado, April 18, 2002.

9. Klempner MS, Hu LT, Evans J, et al. Two controlled trials of antibiotic treatment in patients with persistent symptoms and a history of Lyme disease. N Engl J Med 345:85–92, 2001.

CHAPTER FOURTEEN

HIV–Related Fatigue

Fatigue is a significant problem in the person with human immunodeficiency virus (HIV) infection or acquired immunodeficiency syndrome (AIDS). As with other disorders, the occurrence of fatigue in the HIV/AIDS patient is high, with an estimated frequency of 20% to 60%. The rate of fatigue climbs even higher as the syndrome progresses.[1]

The fatigue associated with HIV is exceptionally important to address, as it can interfere with adherence to antiretroviral therapy regimens that are crucial to viral suppression, and must often be timed precisely. Along with family support, the feeling of an internal locus of control, and such physical effects as pain and numbness in the hands and feet, fatigue is a significant determinant of adherence to antiretroviral therapy.[2] In turn, a successful and well-tolerated antiretroviral regimen contributes significantly to improved quality of life and reduced fatigue.[3]

CAUSES OF FATIGUE

As with any type of fatigue, a number of factors contribute to this symptom in the HIV/AIDS patient, including lack of rest or exercise, improper or inadequate diet, chronic diarrhea, depression and anxiety, low levels of hormones such as testosterone, and anemia (Table 14-1).[1]

Table 14-1. Contributors to Fatigue in the HIV Patient

Lack of rest
Lack of exercise
Improper or inadequate diet
Vitamin deficiency (especially B$_{12}$)
Psychological factors, including depression and anxiety
Use of recreational drugs
Use/abuse of alcohol
Hypothyroidism
Hypogonadism
Infections (acute and chronic)
Side effects of medications
Fever
Sleep disturbances

(Reprinted with permission from Adinolfi A. Assessment and treatment of HIV-related fatigue. J Assoc Nurses AIDS Care 12 [suppl]:29–34, 2001.)

Anemia in particular is a very prominent cause of fatigue in the HIV/AIDS patient. It can result from several factors, including infection, HIV–related cancers (and chemotherapy related to cancer treatment), deficiencies in iron and vitamin B_{12}, and absolute iron deficiency from multiple blood drawing.[4] There is also *treatment-related anemia,* which is related directly to the use of antiretroviral medications. Drugs of the reverse transcriptase inhibitor and protease inhibitor classes can cause severe myelosuppression, and this form of anemia is very difficult to correct.

Infection is a significant contributor to fatigue in HIV/AIDS. The acute infectious phase of HIV itself, when the virus is multiplying rapidly, can cause fatigue symptoms. HIV infection also puts the patient at risk for opportunistic infections, such as pneumonia, that can cause fatigue symptoms in their acute phase and weaken the patient over the long term. Chronic infections such as hepatitis C are also well-known contributors to fatigue, as are parasitic infections of the digestive system, which can cause chronic diarrhea and interfere with nutrient absorption.

Lack of exercise takes a substantial toll on the strength of the HIV patient, leading to fatigue and tiredness. The fatigue of deconditioning can be compounded by the fatigue of anemia and the fatigue that comes from the inability to sustain adequate nutrition. (See Chapter 17 for recommendations regarding nutrition and exercise for fatigue.)

Sleep disturbance has been reported in HIV patients and may be associated with fatigue. In one study of 100 women with HIV or AIDS, those with high levels of fatigue had significantly more difficulty falling asleep, more awakenings from nighttime sleep, poorer daytime functioning, and a higher frequency of depressive symptoms.[5]

Among HIV/AIDS patients, the term *battle fatigue* has been used, and this accurately represents the toll taken by years of coping with a fatal illness and having to adhere precisely to a lifelong demanding antiretroviral medication regimen. Patients who were once expected to have a limited life span are now finding themselves being able to maintain their long-term health, but only through vigilant and aggressive medication use.[6] The psychological consequences of prolonged illness also include depression and anxiety, both of which are associated with fatigue.

MANAGEMENT

Management of fatigue in the HIV/AIDS patient must be multifactorial, addressing nutritional and conditioning concerns, treating opportunistic infections, and finding an antiretroviral therapy regimen that maximizes HIV suppression but minimizes the risks of anemia and liver toxicity. Anemia should be suspected in all HIV/AIDS patients with fatigue, and hemoglobin and hematocrit levels should be routinely checked. Treatments include the use of recombinant human erythropoietin, which stimulates red blood cell production. Although blood transfusion and iron supplementation are also options, there is evidence that blood transfusion can activate HIV expression,[4] and iron supplements often cause gastrointestinal distress and are poorly absorbed.

Few studies have addressed pharmacologic therapies for fatigue in HIV. A recent study found significant improvement in fatigue with testosterone therapy in those who had symptomatic HIV disease and clinical hypogonadism. In this 12-week, 72-patient trial, 79% of those who completed the study responded with improved energy levels and significantly decreased fatigue as measured by the Chalder Fatigue Scale.[7]

Another trial compared the use of the stimulant medications methylphenidate and pemoline with placebo in HIV. The 144 patients in this study were all ambulatory, and were classified as having severe and persistent fatigue. They were randomized to methylphenidate, 60 mg; pemoline, 150 mg; or placebo. Of the 109 patients who completed the trial, 41% of those receiving methylphenidate and 36% of those receiving pemoline reported clinically significant improvement with fatigue on the Piper Fatigue Scale and Visual Analog Scale for Fatigue, compared with 15% of placebo patients. The two drugs performed equally well. Severe side effects were uncommon, and adverse effects overall were of the type generally associated with stimulant medications, including jitteriness.[8]

If there is a significant depressive component to the fatigue, antidepressant therapy may be helpful. Because of the multiple medications that HIV/AIDS patients take, care must be taken to choose an anti-depressant with a low risk of drug-drug interactions.

CONCLUSION

Fatigue in HIV is a multifactorial symptom that is related to the drugs taken for HIV, underlying depression, and the toll taken by years of battling a chronic, ultimately fatal disease that requires the patient to adhere to complicated medication regimens. The fatigue workup in the HIV patients should include an assessment of the impact of all of these factors. There is evidence that testosterone replacement therapy and psychostimulants are both effective for treating HIV-related fatigue, and their use should be considered.

HIV–Related Fatigue: Key Concepts

- Fatigue in HIV is related to physical factors (e.g., the side effects of medications used to treat the infection) and psychological factors (e.g., depression and the mental exhaustion that comes from battling a chronic illness). It is critical to identify fatigue in the HIV–positive patient, as it may interfere with the patient's adherence to anti-HIV therapy.
- The acute infectious phase of HIV can cause fatigue symptoms. In patients in the chronic phase of HIV infection, opportunistic infections such as pneumonia can further weaken the patient and cause fatigue.
- Management of fatigue in the HIV patient should include a nutrition program (see Chapter 17) to maintain strength and prevent HIV wasting. Hemoglobin and hematocrit should be checked for anemia. Psychological factors such as depression should be addressed. Testosterone therapy and psychostimulants may both be effective for reducing the severity of fatigue.

REFERENCES

1. Adinolfi A. Assessment and treatment of HIV-related fatigue. J Assoc Nurses AIDS Care 12 (suppl):29–34, 2001.
2. Molassiotis A, Nahas-Lopez V, Chung WY, et al. Factors associated with adherence to antiretroviral

medication in HIV-infected patients. Int J STD AIDS 13:301–310, 2002.

3. Nieuwkerk PT, Gisolf EH, Reijers MH, et al. Long-term quality of life outcomes in three antiretroviral treatment strategies for HIV-1 infection. AIDS 19:1985–1991, 2001.

4. Moyle G. Anaemia in persons with HIV infection: prognostic marker and contributor to mortality. AIDS Rev 4:13–20, 2002.

5. Lee KA, Portillo CJ, Miramontes H. The influence of sleep and activity patterns on fatigue in women with HIV/AIDS. J Assoc Nurses AIDS Care 12(suppl):19–27, 2001.

6. Farthing CF. Many patients suffer from "battle fatigue": survey. AIDS Alert 16:73–77, 2001.

7. Wagner GJ, Rabkin JG, Rabkin R. Testosterone as a treatment for fatigue in HIV+ men. Gen Hosp Psychiatry 20:209–213, 1998.

8. Breitbart W, Rosenfeld B, Kaim M, Funesti-Esch J. A randomized, double-blind, placebo-controlled trial of psychostimulants for the treatment of fatigue in ambulatory patients with human immunodeficiency virus disease. Arch Intern Med 161:411–420, 2001.

Chronic Fatigue Syndrome

Few disease states have engendered as much controversy in recent years as chronic fatigue syndrome (CFS). A syndrome characterized by the presence of unexplained, persistent recurrent fatigue and a number of nonspecific symptoms including tender lymph nodes, joint and muscle pain, and swelling, CFS has been the object of skepticism among many physicians and strenuous advocacy among patient groups.

The concept of a chronic fatiguing disease state is far from new. Concepts of nonspecific, "enfeebling" diseases of the nervous system (e.g., neurasthenia) can be dated back to the mid-19th century.[1] Findings of asthenia were attributed to chronic fatigue, depression, and even a masculine form of hysteria. Almost from the time this concept of chronic fatigue was introduced, physicians have wrestled with the contrast between the reported degree of physical disability and the lack of consistent, objectively measurable signs or symptoms of disease.[1,2]

The codification of a definition for CFS in 1994 (Box 15-1) has done much to improve research on CFS as a legitimate syndrome.[3] The ultimate Centers for Disease Control and Prevention (CDC) definition was the culmination of a number of published case definitions that had been introduced in the late 1980s and early 1990s.[4–6] Under the case definition that was adopted by the CDC in 1994, the patient must have persistent or recurrent fatigue that results in a substantial impairments in social, occupational, educational, or personal functioning, in addition to at least four of a list of symptoms persisting for at least 6 months.[3]

The lack of specificity of CFS symptomatology is a major challenge both to physicians, who want to give patients the correct answers for their illness, and for patients, who may be struggling to convince physicians (as well as family members, employers, and others) that the illness they have is genuine. The problem is complicated by the heterogeneity of the population; estimates have put the prevalence of CFS at approximately 3% of the primary care population.[7,8]

Box 15-1. Chronic Fatigue Syndrome Diagnostic Criteria

1. Clinically evaluated, unexplained persistent or relapsing chronic fatigue that is of new or definite onset (i.e., not life-long), is not the result of ongoing exertion, is not substantially alleviated by rest, and results in a substantial reduction in previous levels of occupational, educational, social, or personal activities.

2. The concurrent occurrence of four or more of the following symptoms. These symptoms must have persisted or recurred during 6 or more consecutive months, and must not have predated the fatigue:
   - Substantial impairment in short-term memory or concentration
   - Sore throat
   - Tender lymph nodes
   - Muscle pain
   - Multijoint pain without swelling or redness
   - Headaches of a new type, pattern, or severity
   - Unrefreshing sleep
   - Postexertional malaise lasting more than 24 hours

(Source: Fukuda K, Straus SE, Hickie I, et al. The chronic fatigue syndrome: a comprehensive approach to its definition and study. International Fatigue Syndrome Study Group. Ann Intern Med 121:953–959, 1994.

EXPLORING THE CAUSES OF CFS

The investigations into the potential causes of CFS have been distinctive in their inability to identify a discrete cause for CFS. Chronic fatigue syndrome has been attributed, at various times and by various researchers, to infectious disease, neuroendocrine abnormalities, immune dysfunction, and psychiatric illness. Research has implicated dysfunction of the hypothalamic-pituitary-adrenal (HPA) axis (the pathophysiology of which is discussed in more detail in Chapter 5) as playing at least a partial role.[9] Other research has explored the role of autonomic nervous system dysfunction (i.e., neurally mediated hypotension), noting that CFS patients bear some similarities to those with orthostatic hypotension.[10,11]

Of potential infectious causes, the greatest degree of attention has been focused on Epstein-Barr virus (EBV); however, the data accumulated has not supported a causative role for EBV in CFS, and it has been declared unlikely that EBV is the cause.[12] Other investigations into infection with enteroviruses (e.g., coxsackie, poliovirus) and human herpesvirus-6 have been unconvincing.[1]

A variety of immunologic studies have also been conducted in CFS, exploring the potential etiologic role of CD lymphocytes,[13] natural killer cell activity,[14] and cytokines such as interleukin-1, interleukin-6, and tumor necrosis factor-α.[15,16] Although abnormalities have been found, they are neither consistent nor severe enough to provide a satisfactory explanation for CFS symptoms. Furthermore, immune abnormalities do not provide the necessary degree of specificity for a CFS diagnosis.

Other avenues of investigation have been explored, including chemical intolerance to low levels of environmental chemicals,[17] and brain abnormalities on imaging. Studies involving anatomic imaging (e.g., magnetic resonance imaging) and functional imaging (e.g., positron-emission tomography) have found white-matter abnormalities, as well as perfusion defects in certain areas of the frontal and temporal lobes.[18] Imaging for CFS, however, remains largely a research tool.

The lack of consistent biological correlates naturally leads to the question of the potential role of psychological contributors to CFS. Again, the literature here is often inconsistent. As discussed in Chapter 4 and throughout this text, affective disorders, including depression and anxiety, are well-established contributors to fatigue across a number of disease states, and it has been observed that the majority of CFS patients meet lifetime criteria for depression.[19] Investigations have shown a significant degree of association between psychiatric morbidity and unexplained chronic fatigue.[20] CFS is also associated with other clinical conditions with somatic aspects, including fibromyalgia and irritable bowel syndrome.[21] In an epidemiologic study of Baltimore residents who were interviewed at baseline and followed for 13 years, the number of somatization symptoms, along with a history of a dysphoric episode at baseline, were the two strongest predictors of new onset fatigue, as well as recurrent or chronic fatigue.[22]

Various investigators have evaluated the effect of prior physical or sexual abuse on chronic fatigue, concluding that a childhood sexual abuse history may be a predictor of chronic fatigue and other psychiatric disorders (e.g., anxiety, post-traumatic stress syndrome) within chronic fatigue.[23,24]

The patient's attributional qualities may also play a role in CFS symptomatology. It has been reported that, in contrast to patients with depression, whose symptoms were distinguished by low self-esteem and the propensity to make cognitive distortions across situations, CFS patients demonstrate a strong illness identity, external attributions for their illness, and distortions in thinking that are specific to somatic experiences.[19] These illness beliefs can have a profound effect on the way patients approach their illness, the attribution of the causes, and even the outcomes of interventions.[1]

TREATMENT APPROACHES

The treatment studies in CFS have been as varied as the search for an etiology. Various approaches have been aimed at correcting dysregulation of the sympathetic nervous system,[25] use of immunoglobulin,[26] use of corticosteroids[27] or growth hormone,[28] and cognitive behavioral therapy.[29] The studies have employed a number of outcomes, including psychological (anxiety, cognitive functioning, depression, coping strategies); physical (activity, disability, and fatigue); quality of life (employment, patient satisfaction), and physiologic (immunologic outcomes, temperature).[30]

In a systematic review of 44 controlled trials of CFS, the only interventions that showed consistently promising results were cognitive behavioral therapy and graded exercise therapy.[30] (General considerations for exercise therapy and nutrition are discussed in Chapter 17.) Positive outcomes were reported for other therapies (e.g., hydrocortisone, selegeline, essential fatty acids) in various studies. However, conclusions in evaluating overall positive treatment effects were made difficult by the fact that many interventions have been evaluated in only one or two studies, and the studies employed a wide variety of outcome measures and inclusion/exclusion criteria, and some treatments (e.g., hydrocortisone) were associated with unacceptable adverse effects.

CONCLUSION

Research in CFS has greatly added to our knowledge on fatigue in general. Unfortunately, it is unlikely that a set of discrete identifying factors shedding light on the cause of CFS will emerge at any time in the near future. Nevertheless, although the results of studies on various biologic factors as the causes of CFS have not been particularly enlightening, the fact that they have been so aggressively explored is understandable given that CFS patients may still be referred to at times as lazy or psychosomatic.[31] As with all fatigue states, it is important to listen carefully to and acknowledge the patient's complaints of fatigue. Even if a specific biologic cause cannot be identified, it is apparent that something is contributing to the patient's fatigue, and the potential contribution of psychological factors and somatoform disorders are no less important to address, diagnose, and manage fully.[9]

Chronic Fatigue Syndrome: Key Concepts

- Under the case definition for chronic fatigue syndrome (CFS) developed by the Centers for Disease Control and Prevention, the patient must have persistent or recurrent fatigue that results in substantial impairment in social, occupational, educational, or personal functioning, as well as a number of physical symptoms that persist for at least 6 months.

(continued)

Chronic Fatigue Syndrome: Key Concepts—Cont'd

- HPA-axis dysfunction, autonomic nervous system dysfunction, viral infection, immune deficiency, psychological illness, and exposure to chemical contaminants have all been offered at various times to explain the occurrence of CFS. None of these causes, however, can sufficiently account for CFS.
- Persons with CFS tend to demonstrate a strong illness identity and external attributions for their illness.
- The only treatments shown to be consistently beneficial in CFS are graded exercise therapy and cognitive behavioral therapy. Other therapies that have been tried, including immunoglobulin, corticosteroids, and growth hormone, have either been inconsistent in their effects or associated with a high risk of adverse effects.
- Even if a specific biologic basis cannot be identified, the physician must listen carefully to and acknowledge the patient's fatigue. Specific factors to examine that may help explain CFS include the existence of an affective disorder or a somatoform disorder. If these are suspected, it is important to address them fully.

REFERENCES

1. Wessely S, Hotopf M, Sharpe M. Chronic Fatigue and its Syndromes. London: Oxford University Press, 1999.
2. Blocq P. Neurasthenia. Brain 14:306–314, 1894.
3. Fukuda K, Straus SE, Hickie I, et al. The chronic fatigue syndrome: a comprehensive approach to its definition and study. International Fatigue Syndrome Study Group. Ann Intern Med 121:953–959, 1994.
4. Holmes GP, Kaplan JE, Gantz NM, et al. Chronic fatigue syndrome: a working case definition. Ann Intern Med 108:387–389, 1988.
5. Lloyd AR, Wakefield D, Boughton C, Dwyer J. Prevalence of chronic fatigue syndrome in an Australian population. Med J Aust 153:522–528, 1990.
6. Sharpe MC, Archard LC, Bantvala JE, et al. A report—chronic fatigue syndrome: guidelines for research. J R Soc Med 84:118–121, 1991.
7. Wessely S. The epidemiology of chronic fatigue syndrome. Epidemiol Rev 17:139–151, 1995.
8. Demitrack MA. Neuroendocrine aspects of chronic fatigue syndrome: a commentary. Am J Med 105:11S–14S, 1998.
9. Demitrack MA. Neuroendocrine correlates of chronic fatigue syndrome: a brief review. J Psychiatr Res 31:69–82, 1997.
10. DeBecker P. Autonomic testing in chronic fatigue syndrome patients. Am J Med 105(3A): 22S–26S, 1998.
11. Rowe PC, Calkins H. Neurally mediated hypotension and chronic fatigue syndrome. Am J Med 105(3A): 15S–21S, 1998.

12. Schooley R. Epstein-Barr virus. Curr Opin Infect Dis 2:267–271, 1989.

13. Barker A, Fujimura S, Fadem M, et al. Immunologic abnormalities associated with chronic fatigue syndrome. Clin Infect Dis 18(suppl 1): S136–S141, 1994.

14. Peakman M, Deale A, Field R, et al. Clinical improvement in chronic fatigue syndrome is not associated with lymphocyte subsets of function or activation. Clin Immunol Immunopath 82: 83–91, 1997.

15. Vollmer-Conna U, Lloyd A, Hickie I, Wakefield D. Chronic fatigue syndrome: an immunologic perspective. Aust NZ J Psychiatry 32:523–527, 1998.

16. Chao C, Gallagher M, Phair J, Peterson P. Serum neopterin and interleukin 6 levels in chronic fatigue syndrome. J Infect Dis 162:1412–1413, 1990.

17. Bell IR, Baldwin CM, Schwartz GE. Illness from low levels of environmental chemicals: relevance to chronic fatigue syndrome and fibromyalgia. Am J Med 105(3A):74S–82S, 1998.

18. Lange G, Wang S, DeLuca J, Natelson BH. Neuroimaging in chronic fatigue syndrome. Am J Med 105(3A):50S–53S, 1998.

19. Moss-Morris R, Petrie KJ. Discriminating between chronic fatigue syndrome and depression: a cognitive analysis. Psychol Med 31:469–479, 2001.

20. Skapinakis P, Lewis G, Meltzer H. Clarifying the relationship between unexplained chronic fatigue and psychiatric morbidity: results from a community survey in Great Britain. Am J Psychiatry 157:1492–1498, 2000.

21. Aaron LA, Herrell R, Ashton S, et al. Comorbid clinical conditions in chronic fatigue: a co-twin control study. J Gen Intern Med 16:24–31, 2001.

22. Addington AM, Gallo JJ, Ford DE, Eaton WW. Epidemiology of unexplained fatigue and major depression in the community: the Baltimore ECA follow-up, 1981–1994. Psychol Med 31: 1037–1044, 2001.

23. Taylor RR, Jason LA. Sexual abuse, physical abuse, chronic fatigue, and chronic fatigue syndrome: a community-based study. J Nerv Ment Dis 189:709–715, 2001.

24. Taylor RR, Jason LA. Chronic fatigue, abuse-related traumatization, and psychiatric disorders in a community-based sample. Soc Sci Med 55: 247–256, 2002.

25. Natelson BH, Cheu J, Pareja J, et al. Randomized, double-blind, controlled placebo phase in trial of low-dose phenelzine in the chronic fatigue syndrome. Psychopharmacology 124:226–230, 1996.

26. Rowe KS. Double-blind randomized controlled trial to assess the efficacy of intravenous gamma globulin for the management of fatigue of chronic fatigue syndrome in adolescents. J Psychiatr Res 31:133–147, 1997.

27. Cleare AJ, Heap E, Malhi GS, et al. Low-dose hydrocortisone in chronic fatigue syndrome: a randomized crossover trial. Lancet 353:455–458, 1999.

28. Moorkens G, Wynants H, Abs R. Effect of growth hormone treatment in patients with chronic fatigue syndrome: a preliminary study. Growth Horm IGF Res 8:131–133, 1998.

29. Friedberg F, Krupp LB. A comparison of cognitive behavioral treatment for chronic fatigue syndrome and primary depression. Clin Infect Dis 18(suppl 1): S105–S110, 1994.

30. Whiting P, Bagnall AM, Sowden AJ, et al. Interventions for the treatment and management of chronic fatigue syndrome: a systematic review. JAMA 286: 1360–1368, 2001.

31. Kahn MF. Chronic fatigue syndrome: new developments. Joint Bone Spine 67:359–361, 2000.

Chronic Obstructive Pulmonary Disease

Chronic obstructive pulmonary disease (COPD) includes several diseases characterized by chronic airflow obstruction that is, at best, partially reversible. These include chronic bronchitis, emphysema, and a chronic obstructive form of asthma. The airflow obstruction and permanent lung damage that these patients experience is at the heart of fatigue. COPD patients have spirometric measures that fall well below those for normal persons in terms of forced expiratory volume in 1 second (FEV_1) and forced vital capacity. They also have decreased oxygen saturation, meaning that they have poor oxygen delivery to muscles for use as energy. Add to these the fact that most COPD patients are older, having contracted the disease after decades of smoking and years of deconditioning caused by an inability to sustain aerobic activity, it is not surprising that fatigue is a major part of daily life for most COPD patients.

In stable COPD patients (i.e., those not experiencing exacerbations), dyspnea, wheezing, and physical activity, and fatigue have been shown to be significantly intercorrelated in the COPD patient, with higher dyspnea scores yielding higher fatigue scores.[1] COPD patients also experience periodic exacerbations, which may weaken the patient and cause infection, increasing fatigue through deconditioning, further oxygen desaturation, and the general stress response.

Depression is common in COPD, as are anxiety disorders. Although the link between COPD, anxiety, and depression has not been systematically explored, the relationship between these three factors in other disorders certainly suggests that an association is plausible in COPD.

As with many fatiguing disorders, underlying sleep disturbances may play a significant role in fatigue in the COPD patient. Poor sleep may result from a number of causes, including cough, excess mucus production, and frequent arousals from hypercapnia.[2] While benzodiazepines can be used to improve sleep, they should be used with caution in the COPD patient as they can cause a reduction in upper airway muscle tone.

MANAGEMENT

The first step in treating fatigue in the COPD patient is careful management of the underlying symptoms of dyspnea with appropriate medications, including β_2 agonists and anticholinergic bronchodilators. These can help prevent exacerbations and subsequent infection, which may lead to respiratory crisis.

The management of COPD symptoms has benefited from the widespread adoption of comprehensive pulmonary rehabilitation programs. Such facilities approach the issue of COPD education in a multidisciplinary fashion, offering tailored exercise programs, weight training, and means to improve breathing (i.e., through maintaining exhalation tension by purse-lipped breathing). The American Lung Association (www.lungusa.org) can be helpful in finding a local pulmonary rehabilitation program for the patient.

Pulmonary rehabilitation programs are of immense benefit for improving strength and treating symptoms in patients with severe COPD.[3] However, they are also effective for reducing symptoms of fatigue and dyspnea even in those with mild stage disease, as measured by increases in treadmill time and 6-minute walks.[4] Long-term trials of rehabilitation programs that include breathing retraining and chest physiotherapy have shown that health-related quality of life can be improved over several years.[3] These programs have also been shown to decrease muscle fatigability in the quadriceps muscle in COPD patients.[5]

Acute oxygen supplementation improves peak exercise capacity and relieve performance fatigue.[6] In a group of 14 patients with FEV_1 levels that were 35% of predicted, administration of oxygen (FiO_2 of 0.75), resulted in an improvement in peak leg exercise capacity. Notably, oxygen is the only intervention that has been shown to prolong life in the COPD patient.

COPD and Fatigue: Key Concepts

- The irreversible lung damage caused by chronic obstructive pulmonary disease (COPD) causes severe decreases in lung function and oxygen utilization. These, in combination with the increased demands on the respiratory muscles, can easily lead to fatigue. Spirometry can be performed easily during the patient visit to test for decreased lung capacity and the possibility of COPD.

(continued)

COPD and Fatigue: Key Concepts—Cont'd

- In the stable COPD patient, dyspnea and wheezing are associated with higher levels of fatigue. These symptoms should be controlled using β_2 agonist bronchodilators and anticholinergic inhalers, as well as oxygen therapy.
- COPD exacerbations can cause fatigue by weakening patients, putting them at risk for infection, and increasing the body's stress response.
- Depression, anxiety, and sleep disturbances are all common in COPD patients. A course of antidepressant therapy may help alleviate depression and anxiety symptoms. Managing symptoms of cough and excessive mucus production can improve sleep.
- Deconditioning is a major cause of fatigue in the COPD patient. Pulmonary rehabilitation should be considered essential in COPD patients to maintain aerobic capacity and muscle strength. The American Lung Association (www.lungusa.org) can be helpful in finding a pulmonary rehabilitation program for a patient.

REFERENCES

1. Woo K. A pilot study to examine the relationships of dyspnoea, physical activity and fatigue in patients with chronic obstructive pulmonary disease. J Clin Nurs 9:526–533, 2000.

2. George CF. Perspectives on the management of insomnia in patients with chronic respiratory disorders. Sleep 23(suppl 1):S31–S35, 2000.

3. Guell R, Casan P, Belda J, et al. Long-term effects of outpatient rehabilitation of COPD: a randomized trial. Chest 117:976–983, 2000.

4. Berry MJ, Rejeski WJ, Adair NE, Zaccaro D. Exercise rehabilitation and chronic obstructive pulmonary disease stage. Am J Respir Crit Care Med 160:1248–1253, 1999.

5. Mador MJ, Kufel TJ, Pineda LA, et al. Effect of pulmonary rehabilitation on quadriceps fatiguability during exercise. Am J Respir Crit Care Med 163:930–935, 2001.

6. Maltais F, Simon M, Jobin J, et al. Effects of oxygen on lower limb blood flow and O_2 uptake during exercise in COPD. Med Sci Sports Exerc 33:916–922, 2001.

PART THREE

Fatigue Management

Treatment Approaches

Given the significant heterogeneity of fatigue and the wide variety of disorders in which fatigue can present, it is difficult to make universal recommendations regarding treatment approaches. More research has been conducted in some fatiguing disease states than in others, and it is difficult to predict whether an approach that has been effective for fatigue in one type of disorder (e.g., multiple sclerosis [MS]) will translate into an effective treatment for another disorder (e.g., chronic fatigue syndrome [CFS]). This chapter focuses on some of the treatments for which there is empiric support in the literature.

As with any symptom, an effective fatigue treatment plan begins with a comprehensive assessment and diagnostic protocol. As discussed in Chapter 3, there are several fatigue scales that can be used to assess the presence and severity of fatigue, and pointed questions about the onset of fatigue and surrounding circumstances (e.g., stress in work and family situations) provide important guidance on the types of treatment that may be most beneficial.

A COMPREHENSIVE TREATMENT PLAN

The treatment plan for the fatigued patient should always begin with education on fatigue. In cases in which fatigue will be expected in the future (e.g., after surgery or during chemotherapy), patients should be told beforehand what to expect and asked to keep close track of their energy levels. In patients who already have fatigue by the time they reach the physician's office, the physician should explain the potential causes of fatigue and discuss with them what can be done. The primary point to stress is that, although fatigue may be a natural symptom of any disease or disorder, it can be treated effectively.

Education should extend to the patient's family and/or significant other as well. This will help the family understand what is happening to the patient, and begin to get them involved in planning to ease physical and mental burdens that may be contributing to the patient's fatigue. It will also help to clear up misperceptions (e.g., that the patient is simply lazy).

Nutrition/Dietary Interventions

Patients should be given a comprehensive assessment of their nutritional intake and referred for consultation with a nutritionist, if possible. Although there is no particular diet or dietary supplement (with the exception of iron in anemia states) that will reduce fatigue, adherence to a balanced nutritional program will help maintain overall health and strength. Boxes 17-1 and 17-2 outline some tips for nutritional interventions. For patients who have trouble taking in sufficient calories to maintain their strength (e.g., HIV patients and cancer patients undergoing chemotherapy), good nutrition should not be sacrificed, but the overriding goal is to ensure that enough total calories are being consumed.

Energy Conservation Strategies

Although energy conservation strategies have not been examined through clinical trials, they have become a widespread means of helping those with moderate-to-severe fatigue accomplish activities of daily living and remain active. Strategies, outlined in Box 17-3, are designed to make tasks such as meal

---

Box 17-1. Nutritional Interventions for Fatigue

There is no single type of diet or food that specifically treats fatigue. However, patients should always be educated on the basics of good nutrition program. These include:

- **Drink enough water:** Everyone should drink at least eight 8-ounce glasses of water every day. Dehydration can intensify fatigue.

- **Avoid sugars and sweets, especially refined sugars:** These can cause changes in blood glucose levels. The spike and then sharp drop in blood glucose after sugar is consumed can lead to tiredness.

- **Make every meal count:** Eat high-nutrient, high-protein, complex carbohydrate foods.

- **Reduce portion sizes and eat more often:** Eat smaller meals throughout the day instead of three large meals. This will help stabilize energy levels throughout the day. Large meals also make the patient feel tired and lethargic.

- **Eat a high-protein meal in the morning:** A high-protein meal in the morning may increase productivity and energy. In the evening, a small meal that is higher in complex carbohydrates can help produce serotonin, which has relaxing effects.

- **Eat complex carbohydrates:** Starches such as potatoes and sweet potatoes are well-tolerated carbohydrates that are easy to digest and contain high amounts of vitamins A and C.

- **Eat legumes:** Beans and peas are high in complex carbohydrates, which regulates blood sugar levels. They are also high in iron, zinc, and B vitamins.

- **Increase fruit and vegetable intake:** Vegetables are high in calcium, magnesium, and potassium, as well as antioxidants including vitamins A and C. Fruits are also high in vitamins, and both are high in fiber, which can avoid constipation.

(continued)

Box 17-1. Nutritional Interventions for Fatigue—Cont'd

- **Eat foods high in iron:** If iron-deficiency anemia is suspected, eat foods that are high in iron, such as red meat, leafy green vegetables, and iron-fortified cereals.
- **Avoid caffeine:** This is especially important later in the day. Caffeine acts like a central nervous system stimulant and can interfere with sleep.
- **Avoid tobacco and alcohol:** Tobacco and alcohol also act as stimulants, and can interfere with sleep. Alcohol is also an empty source of calories.
- **Exercise regularly:** Regular exercise can help stimulate the appetite.
- **Eat to maintain a healthy weight:** Carrying extra weight increases stress on the body. If you are overweight, a reduced-fat, balanced diet should be followed.
- **Be cautious of supplements and herbal remedies:** Various supplements and herbal remedies have been proposed to help fatigue, but with the exception of iron supplementation for anemia, there is no evidence that these supplements are beneficial. The best way to receive vitamins and minerals is through foods; however, a multivitamin may be recommended.

Box 17-2. Nutritional Interventions for Fatigue

For the patient who has trouble maintaining weight (e.g., cancer patients undergoing chemotherapy, those with HIV-wasting disease, and those with prolonged mobility restrictions after

(continued)

Box 17-2. Nutritional Interventions for Fatigue—Cont'd

surgery), it is essential to consume enough calories to provide the body with the energy it needs. Some strategies include:

- **Aim for foods with high-calorie content:** Eating high-calorie foods such as ice cream and commercially available liquid nutritional drinks can help ensure that the patient gets adequate calories.
- **Choose enjoyable foods:** Cold, smooth foods such as frozen yogurt, ice cream, or a fruit smoothie can make eating more enjoyable when the patient's appetite is low.
- **Limit liquids during mealtime:** Drinking water or other liquids during a meal may make the patient feel more full. The patient can drink after or an hour or so before the meal.
- **Be prepared:** Suggest that the patient keep a stock of easy-to-prepare foods, such as frozen dinners or canned soups.
- **Take advantage of hunger:** Many individuals have larger appetites in the morning. The patient can take advantage of this by eating a large breakfast and treating breakfast as the main meal of the day.
- **Think ahead:** On days on which fatigue is more tolerable and the patient feels like cooking, he or she can make extra portions and freeze the rest in individual serving containers.
- **Stimulate the appetite:** A number of medications, such as selective serotonin reuptake inhibitors (SSRIs), act as appetite stimulators and can help the patient maintain weight. Consider using them, especially in patients who also have depression or anxiety.
- **Ask for help:** Remind the patient that he or she does not have to endure fatigue alone. Family and friends can be called on to cook and bring over meals.

Box 17-3. Energy Conservation Strategies

There are a number of energy-saving tips that can help the fatigue patient maintain their activities of daily living. Some include:

- **Plan for higher-energy periods:** The patient should accomplish more difficult tasks (e.g., grocery shopping) when fatigue feels least severe. Keeping a daily fatigue diary for a week or two can help the patient recognize the times of day when fatigue may be less severe.
- **Build in rest periods:** Taking short rests (10 or 15 minutes) throughout the day can help maintain energy. The patient should avoid excessive napping, which may interfere with nighttime sleep.
- **Maintain a regular sleep schedule:** Sleeping regular hours and avoiding unnecessary late nights can avoid fluctuations in energy levels throughout the day.
- **Plan ahead and pace activities:** Patients can make daily or weekly schedules of activities and pace their activities, taking short rest periods during prolonged activity (e.g., work).
- **Postpone nonessential activities:** Emphasize to the patient that it is OK to postpone activities that are not absolutely essential when their fatigue is moderate to severe. This may help alleviate guilt in patients who feel they need to accomplish everything.
- **Engage in "restorative" activities:** Activities such as meditation, yoga, sitting in the park, and walking on the beach can have a restorative influence on patients, helping them feel more balanced and energetic, and reducing stress.

(continued)

Box 17-3. Energy Conservation Strategies—Cont'd

- **Rearrange the home to fight fatigue:** Placing items in strategic locations can help reduce energy expenditures. For example, putting cleaning products in the upstairs, as well as downstairs rooms can avoid multiple trips up and down the stairs.
- **Get everyone involved:** The patient should get family and friends involved in strenuous activities such as laundry, housecleaning, and yard work. The physician explaining this to the family may help ensure their assistance.
- **Think of alternative ways to accomplish things:** Daily or weekly errands can be made easier. For example, patients may be surprised to find out that many grocery stores still deliver upon request. Most banks will also take deposits by mail, avoiding a trip to the bank. If the patient has a computer, many agencies (for example, departments of motor vehicles) have forms on the Internet that can minimize the time spent standing in line and filling out forms. Remind the patient that it never hurts to check.

---

preparation, shopping, and daily errands easier. Consultation with an occupational therapist may be helpful.

Exercise Programs

Exercise regimens that are tailored within the patient's level of physical ability are of obvious benefit for their overall effects on aerobic functioning and strength. Regardless of the patient's underlying disease and the reason for fatigue, an exercise plan should be made part of any overall wellness plan unless there is some clear contraindication to exercise therapy (e.g., advanced cardiac disease).

Exercise programs have been studied in several disorders in which fatigue is a symptom, including multiple sclerosis (MS), cancer, and chronic obstructive pulmonary disease (COPD).[1-4] Benefits have been seen in exercise endurance,[1,2] as well as improvement on specific measures of fatigue, including the fatigue subscale of the Profile of Mood States (POMS).[3] Exercise may also be beneficial in helping to upregulate cortisol levels, which are implicated in fatigue pathophysiology, and may be chronically low in states of deconditioning (see Chapter 5). Some exercise recommendations are outlined in Box 17-4.

Psychological Interventions

Several randomized, controlled trials have evaluated cognitive behavioral therapy (CBT) in chronic fatigue syndrome (CFS) populations, showing various degrees of long-term benefit. For example, in a 5-year follow-up by Deale et al., of 53 patients who received either CBT or relaxation therapy, 68% of those who received CBT considered themselves

Box 17-4. Exercise Interventions

Exercise can help increase stamina and oxygen utilization by increasing aerobic capacity. It can also strengthen muscles, and increase energy reserves. Endorphins produced by exercise can decrease feelings of depression and anxiety.

Virtually all patients can engage in some form of exercise therapy. The following are some guidelines:

- **Individualize the plan:** The disease or condition underlying the fatigue symptom (e.g., cancer, MS, surgery, Parkinson's disease) can have a marked influence on the approach to exercise therapy. In the postoperative patient, for example, the primary goal should be limited to early postoperative mobilization. For the Parkinson's disease patient with transferring difficulties, a program such as stationary cycling, which presents fewer balance problems, may be more appropriate than walking or jogging. COPD patients, who have severe restrictions on lung capacity, should be referred to a pulmonary rehabilitation center for a specialized program.

- **Start slow and build up:** Starting with a moderate exercise program is essential to avoid undue stress on the body and to promote adherence to the program. Exercise for fatigue has been studied most closely in those with MS and cancer, but the principles can be applied to other fatigue states. Suggestions include the use of a pyramid approach both for muscle fitness and physical activity. For muscle fitness, patients should start with simple range-of-motion exercises, gradually working up to integrated strength training exercises.

For activity, patients should be matched by ability to their functional level, starting by performing as many normal daily

(continued)

Box 17-4. Exercise Interventions—Cont'd

activities as possible. From there, patients can move to more active recreation and eventually a structured exercise program (e.g., walking for 20 minutes a day).

- **Make sure the patient has the right equipment:** Adaptive equipment, such as orthoses, may be needed depending on the patient's level of disability. The physician must make sure that patients with potentially limiting disabilities have the right equipment. Consultation with a physical therapist is recommended.

- **Plan in advance for fatigue:** Patients should make sure they receive adequate sleep the night before exercising and schedule exercise for the time of day when they feel most energetic. Patients should never exercise to the point of exhaustion.

- **Make exercise a prescription:** Giving the patient a sense of accountability for his or her exercise program can help ensure adherence to the program. Make the patient keep an exercise diary that can be discussed with the physician at every visit.

- **Reward performance:** Set a program for patients in which they give themselves "token economies" (small rewards) for achieving exercise goals. For example, patients can reward themselves with a new shirt or pair of shoes for keeping with the program for 2 weeks; 3 months can earn a trip to the theater. Such strategies are especially important with the fatigue patient, who may suffer from lack of motivation or depression along with fatigue.

- **Make it a group effort:** Suggest that the patient find a group to exercise with on a regular basis. This can make exercise more fun and promote adherence to the program.

"much improved" or "very much improved" at the 5-year follow-up point.[5] Approximately one third of those receiving relaxation therapy reported the same levels of improvement.

Such behavioral therapies, along with graded exercise therapy, are the only therapies of proven benefit in the CFS population. In the most comprehensive review of potential fatigue therapies, Whiting et al. examined 44 controlled trials, 36 of which were randomized, and categorized treatment strategies as behavioral (exercise therapy or CBT); immunologic (including immunoglobulin and hydrocortisone); pharmacologic; supplements; complementary/alternative therapies; and other interventions. A total of 2801 patients had participated in the 44 trials. In the results, only CBT and graded exercise therapy showed promising results. Although some limited positive results were seen with immunologic therapies, the findings were inconclusive overall, and there was insufficient evidence with the other four categories.[6]

Pharmacologic Therapies

There are a number of pharmacologic approaches that have been employed to ameliorate fatigue in various diseases (Table 17-1). For fatigue associated specifically with anemia, iron supplementation and exogenous erythropoietin have been shown to improve hemoglobin levels and lessen fatigue.[7]

Agents that have been employed for generalized fatigue include dopaminergic medications, psychostimulants, wake-promoting agents, and antidepressant and antianxiety agents. As discussed in Chapter 7, much of the work with pharmacologic therapy has been performed in the field of MS.[8–10] However, positive results for fatigue and/or hypersomnolence with pharmacologic therapies have been seen in postpolio syndrome (bromocriptine and amantadine)[11,12]; Parkinson's disease (modafinil)[13]; cancer (methylphenidate)[14]; and HIV disease (testosterone replacement, methylphenidate, and pemoline).[15,16]

Among the pharmacologic agents, amantadine has shown promise in several studies of MS patients.[8,17–19] The medication is an antiviral agent that is also believed to act along dopaminergic pathways. It has shown benefits in approximately one third of MS patients. Given its favorable safety profile and the fact that it is inexpensive, it is a worthwhile medication to try in fatigue patients.

There are a number of central nervous system (CNS) stimulants, including pemoline and methylphenidate, which are generally approved for use in the treatment of attention-deficit hyperactivity disorder. These medications act to produce wakefulness along the mesocorticolimbic pathways (the

Table 17-1. Pharmacologic Agents of Potential Benefit for Fatigue*

Drug	Starting Dose	Usual Maintenance Dose	Usual Maximum Dose	Adverse Effects
Amantadine	100 mg q AM or 100 mg bid	100 mg bid	300 mg/d	Livedo reticularis, insomnia
Modafinil	100 mg q AM	200 mg q AM or 100 mg bid	400 mg/d	Headache, insomnia
Pemoline	18.75 mg/d	18.75–55.5 mg/d	93.75 mg/d	Irritability, restlessness, insomnia (?), LFT changes
Recombinant human erythropoietin†	**HIV:** 100 U/kg tiw **Cancer:** 150 U/kg tiw **Surgery:** 300 U/kg tiw for 10 days before surgery, the day of surgery, and for 4 days after surgery	**HIV:** Increase starting dose by 50–100 U/kg tiw until desired effect is seen (hematocrit of 36%) **Cancer:** 150–300 U/kg	**HIV/cancer:** 300 U/kg tiw **Surgery:** N/A	Fever, nausea, constipation
Iron supplementation†	18 mg/d	100 mg/d	200 mg/d	Gastric irritation, blood in stool
Folic acid†	300 µg/d	300–400 µg/d	1000 µg/d	Vitamin B$_{12}$ deficiency (?)

Methylphenidate	**Extended release:** 18 mg/d **Immediate release:** 20–30 mg in divided doses (bid or tid)	**Extended release:** 18–54 mg/d **Immediate release:** 20–30 mg/d	**Extended release:** 54 mg/d **Immediate release:** 60 mg/d	Headache, anorexia, abdominal pain, insomnia
Bupropion (sustained release)	150 mg/d in the AM	150 mg bid	200 mg bid	Agitation, anxiety, insomnia
Fluoxetine	20 mg/d in the AM	20–80 mg/d	80 mg/d	Asthenia, nausea, insomnia
Protriptyline	15 mg/d	15–40 mg/d in 3–4 divided doses	60 mg/d	Seizures, urinary retention, nausea
Bromocriptine	0.5–5 mg bid with food	5 mg bid; increase by 2.5 mg/d if necessary every 14–28 d	100 mg/d	Nausea, hallucinations, confusion
Testosterone replacement‡	50 mg IM q 2–4 wk	50–400 mg q 2–4 wk	400 mg q 2–4 wk	Nausea, gynecomastia, hirsutism, injection-site reactions

*Adult doses given in all cases.

†These agents are recommended for fatigue related to anemia (e.g., cancer, surgery, HIV disease).

‡Testosterone therapy should only be considered in men with HIV disease who have a deficiency of endogenous testosterone.

pathways involved in the vigilance, or "fight or flight" response). The greatest degree of experience with these medications has probably been with pemoline, which has been examined in several trials of MS patients.[8,10] Results of these trials have been mixed, with higher doses (more than 75.5 mg/day) tending to show a limited degree of benefit.[10]

Although these medications may be tried in patients with severe, debilitating fatigue, there are limitations to their use. Methylphenidate and amphetamine are schedule 2 medications, reflecting their potential for abuse. The adverse effects seen with these medications are typical of those seen in the CNS stimulant class, including increases in peripheral autonomic effects (increased heart rate and blood pressure), heightened motor activity, and activation of the brain's "reward system." Thus, they should be used with caution in cases in which long-term use of an agent is expected.

Significant attention has been focused lately on modafinil, an agent that is approved for the treatment of excessive daytime sleepiness associated with narcolepsy. Modafinil is not a stimulant; rather, it is believed to be a unique "wake-promoting" medication that exerts effects through pathways of "normal wakefulness." It has been shown to reduce fatigue scores on the Fatigue Severity Scale (FSS) and several other fatigue scales in MS. Although its use in fatigue in other disease states has not been examined as extensively, it has shown efficacy in reducing hypersomnolence in several disease states, such as Parkinson's disease,[13] depression,[20] and obstructive sleep apnea.[21]

Given the documented association between fatigue, depression, and anxiety, use of antidepressant and/or antianxiety agents may be advantageous in the treatment of fatigue. The benefits for their use in fatigue are largely anecdotal; however, if a patient screening suggests the presence of concomitant depression, a trial of an antidepressant can be given. The selective serotonin reuptake inhibitors (SSRIs) have obvious benefits in terms of their safety profiles, and certain agents (e.g., fluoxetine and venlafaxine), in addition to certain tricyclic antidepressants (e.g., protriptyline), are considered to have "activating properties" that may make them better choices than other antidepressants with more sedating properties. The norepinephrine reuptake inhibitor bupropion is also considered to have activating properties. Antidepressants may also help stimulate the appetite in persons who are not meeting their nutritional needs.

Antianxiety medications are problematic in that most of the traditional agents (e.g., benzodiazepines) have sedating and muscle relaxant effects. Fortunately, in patients for whom anxiety is suspected to contribute to fatigue, the SSRIs have also proven efficacy in anxiety treatment, and several agents in this class are now approved for the treatment of various anxiety disorders, including generalized anxiety disorder. Both antidepressants and antianxiety agents, as well as other medications (e.g., dopamine agonists for restless legs syndrome) may be helpful if it is determined that sleep problems are contributing to daytime fatigue.

CONCLUSION

Regardless of its cause or severity, fatigue should be considered a treatable symptom by the physician. Although the data, especially those on pharmacologic therapies, are generally stronger in certain diseases than in others, the safety of therapies such as modafinil and amantadine, which have been proven effective in MS, make them reasonable choices for other fatiguing disorders, such as cancer, Parkinson's disease, and depression. The benefits of exercise in improving strength, endurance, and mood are nearly universal, and CBT is a reasonable course of treatment for any patient, such as those with CFS or fibromyalgia, who presents with nonspecific fatigue symptoms that are resistant to treatment.

REFERENCES

1. Berry MJ, Rejeski WJ, Adair NE, Zaccaro D. Exercise rehabilitation and chronic obstructive pulmonary disease stage. Am J Respir Crit Care Med 160:1248–1253, 1999.
2. Guell R, Casan P, Belda J, et al. Long-term effects of outpatient rehabilitation of COPD: a randomized trial. Chest 117:976–983, 2000.
3. Petajan JH, Gappmaier E, White AT, et al. Impact of aerobic training on fitness and quality of life in multiple sclerosis. Ann Neurol 39:432–441, 1996.
4. Dimeo FC. Effects of exercise on cancer-related fatigue. Cancer 92:1689–1693, 2001.
5. Deale A, Husain K, Chalder T, Wessely S. Long-term outcome of cognitive behavior therapy versus relaxation therapy for chronic fatigue syndrome: a 5-year follow-up study. Am J Psychiatry 158:2038–2042, 2001.
6. Whiting P, Bagnall AM, Sowden AJ, et al. Interventions for the treatment and management of chronic fatigue syndrome: a systematic review. JAMA 286:1360–1368, 2001.
7. Abels R. Erythropoietin for anemia in cancer patients. Eur J Cancer 29(suppl 2):1616–1634, 1993.
8. Krupp LB, Coyle PK, Doscher C, et al. Fatigue therapy in multiple sclerosis: results of a double-blind, randomized, parallel trial of amantadine, pemoline, and placebo. Neurology 45:1956–1961, 1995.
9. Rammohan KW, Rosenberg JH, Lynn DJ, et al. Efficacy and safety of modafinil (Provigil) for the treatment of fatigue in multiple sclerosis: a

two-centre phase 2 study. J Neurol Neurosurg Psychiatry 72:179–183, 2002.

10. Weinshenker BG, Penman M, Bass B, et al. A double-blind, randomized, crossover trial of pemoline in fatigue associated with multiple sclerosis. Neurology 42:1468–1471, 1992.

11. Bruno RL, Zimmerman JR, Creange SJ, et al. Bromocriptine in the treatment of post-polio fatigue: a pilot study with implications for the pathophysiology of fatigue. Am J Phys Med Rehabil 75:340–347, 1996.

12. Stein DP, Dambrosia JM, Dalakas MC. A double-blind, controlled trial of amantadine for the treatment of fatigue in patients with the post-polio syndrome. Ann NY Acad Sci 25:296–302, 1995.

13. Nieves AV, Lange AE. Treatment of excessive daytime sleepiness in patients with Parkinson's disease with modafinil. Clin Neuropharmacol 25:111–114, 2002.

14. Sarhill N, Walsh D, Nelson KA, et al. Methylphenidate for fatigue advanced cancer: a prospective open-label pilot study. Am J Hosp Palliat Care 18:187–192, 2001.

15. Wagner GJ, Rabkin JG, Rabkin R. Testosterone as a treatment for fatigue in HIV+ men. Gen Hosp Psychiatry 20:209–213, 1998.

16. Breitbart W, Rosenfeld B, Kaim M, Funesti-Esch J. A randomized, double-blind, placebo-controlled trial of psychostimulants for the treatment of fatigue in ambulatory patients with human immunodeficiency virus disease. Arch Intern Med 161:411–420, 2001.

17. Cohen RA, Fisher M. Amantadine treatment of fatigue associated with multiple sclerosis. Arch Neurol 46:676–680, 1989.

18. Murray TJ. Amantadine therapy for fatigue in multiple sclerosis. Can J Neurol Sci 12:251–254, 1985.

19. Canadian MS Research Group. A randomized controlled trial of amantadine in fatigue associated with MS. Can J Neurosci 14:273–279, 1987.

20. Menza MA, Kaufman KR, Castellanos A. Modafinil augmentation of antidepressant treatment in depression. J Clin Psychiatry 61:378–381, 2000.

21. Arnulf I, Homeyer P, Garma L, et al. Modafinil in obstructive sleep apnea-hypopnea syndrome: a pilot study in 6 patients. Respiration 64:159–161, 1997.

CHAPTER EIGHTEEN

Conclusions

I hope that this book has brought the reader some awareness of how common fatigue is in our patient populations, and how difficult it is to identify and treat. Fatigue will continue to be one of the most prevalent problems that physicians encounter, regardless of the area of practice, and it is important to be attuned to the presence of fatigue, to assess its impact on patient well-being, and offer a meaningful treatment plan that is designed to improve functioning and quality of life.

This book provides a guideline for recognizing, assessing, and treating fatigue in a number of disorders. The physician should be aware that there are many other diseases in which fatigue is a symptom, including arthritis, Sjogren's syndrome, fibromyalgia (which has substantial overlap with chronic fatigue syndrome and post-Lyme disease), end-stage renal disease, congestive heart failure, and epilepsy. Therefore, in any disorder, whether chronic or acute, asking initial questions about fatigue/ tiredness is a good strategy.

The many disorders in which fatigue is a symptom and the number of co-occurring factors present almost limitless areas for research, not only for physicians, but also for psychologists, nurses, and rehabilitation providers. Research areas include focusing on a greater understanding of whether fatigue in different disorders has a similar pathophysiologic basis, and if so, whether therapeutic strategies that relieve fatigue in one disease state are able to do so in other diseases.

The end-of-chapter references are one initial source to start for researchers who want to build their library of fatigue literature. The research cited here is by some of the best-known health care providers in their particular fields, and a thorough read of this literature can shed light on the various trial designs that have been conducted, and the interplay of fatigue, depression, anxiety, sleepiness, and other cofactors that can influence treatment outcomes.

Numerous resources are available to the researcher who wishes to conduct a trial on fatigue, including local, regional, and national chapters of disease societies (e.g., the National Multiple Sclerosis

onsortium of Multiple Sclerosis
ie American Parkinson's Disease Asso-
searchers who wish to conduct trials on
ay wish to contact such organizations.
lly the future will bring improved assessment
treatment strategies for severe fatigue.

Index

Page references followed by "f" indicate figures, "t" indicate tables, and "b" indicate boxes.

Abnormal fatigue, 13–14
Abortive polio, 117
Acquired immunodeficiency
    syndrome, 21
    See also Human
    immunodeficiency virus
Adrenal gland, 63
Adrenocorticotropic
    hormone, 63
Alcohol, 211b
Alkaline phosphatase, 86t
Amantadine
    for multiple sclerosis–
    associated fatigue,
    101–103, 102t, 107b,
    219, 220t
    for postpolio
    syndrome–associated
    fatigue, 118–120,
    119b–120b

Aminopyridines, 106
Amyotrophic lateral
    sclerosis, 62
Anemia
    cancer-related fatigue
        caused by,
        134–135, 139
    description of, 21
    human immunodeficiency
        virus–related fatigue
        caused by, 179
    iron-deficiency, 211b
    iron supplementation for,
        220t
    nutritional interventions
        for, 211b
    postoperative, 150b
    systemic lupus
        erythematosus–related
        fatigue and, 163

Anemia—*continued*
   therapies that cause, 179
   treatment of, 139, 150b,
      218–219
Animal models, 73
Antianxiety medications,
   223–224
Antibiotics, for Lyme
   disease–related
   fatigue, 172
Antidepressants, 203b,
   223–224
Antinuclear antibodies, 86t
Appetite stimulators, 212b
Autoimmune disorders,
   65–66
Autonomic nervous system,
   68–69, 73b

Baclofen, 95
Battle fatigue, 180
Beck Depression Inventory, 40
Blood pressure, 68
Blood urea nitrogen, 86t
Borrelia burgdorferi, 169. *See
   also* Lyme disease
Bromocriptine, 118, 119b,
   221t
Bupropion, 221t

Calcium, 86t
Cancer Fatigue Scale, 138–139
Cancer-related fatigue
   anemia, 134–135, 139
   assessment of, 138–139
   causes of, 133–137,
      134t, 141b

   characteristics of, 133
   chemotherapy and, 135
   description of, 20–21, 131
   employment changes
      caused by, 137
   exercise benefits for, 140
   inadequate management
      of, 131, 137–138
   incidence of, 132, 132f
   management of, 137–140
   mental vs. physical fatigue,
      135–136
   onset of, 133
   pain management benefits
      for, 138
   prevalence of, 20t
   quality of life effects,
      132–133
   radiation therapy and, 135
   scales for assessing, 138–139
   summary overview of,
      140–141, 141b
   treatment of, 137–140
   website resources, 133
Categorical view, 13–14
Center for Epidemiologic
   Studies Depression
   Scale, 40
Centers for Disease Control,
   9, 10b, 186, 187b
Central nervous system
   mechanisms, 60–62
Cerebral metabolism
   studies, 93–94
CES-D. *See* Center for
   Epidemiologic Studies
   Depression Scale

CFS. *See* Chronic fatigue
    syndrome
Chemotherapy, 135
Chest examination, 85
Chronic fatigue syndrome
    affective distress in, 50f
    attributional qualities of
        patient and, 190
    blood pressure and, 68
    causes of, 187–190
    Center for Disease Control
        definition of,
        186, 187b
    characteristics of, 185
    cognitive behavioral
        therapy for, 191
    cortisol reductions in, 64
    course of, 63
    definition of, 186, 187b
    depression and, 51
    description of, 9, 22
    diagnostic criteria,
        186, 187b
    Epstein-Barr virus
        and, 188
    fatigue measurements
        in, 31
    history of, 185–186
    hypothalamic-pituitary-
        adrenal axis
        dysfunction and, 188
    immune system
        dysfunction in, 66
    immunologic factors, 188
    infectious causes of, 188
    Lyme disease and, 172
    pain associated with, 49

    post-Lyme disease and, 22
    postpolio syndrome and,
        115–116
    prevalence of, 186
    psychological factors, 189
    sexual abuse and, 190
    somatization symptoms
        and, 69, 189–190
    stressors that affect, 63
    summary overview of,
        191–192, 192b–193b
    treatment of, 190–191
Chronic obstructive pul-
    monary disease
    characteristics of, 199–200
    definition of, 199
    depression and, 200
    dyspnea and, 200
    fatigue associated with
        antidepressants, 203b
        benzodiazepines for,
            200–201
        deconditioning
            and, 203b
        exacerbations, 203b
        management of,
            201–202
        oxygen supplementation
            for, 202
        pulmonary rehabilitation
            programs for,
            201–202
        sleep disturbances and,
            200–201
        summary overview of,
            202b–203b
Cigarette smoking, 83

Cognitive behavioral therapy
for chronic fatigue
syndrome, 191
for depression, 51–52
for multiple sclerosis–
associated fatigue,
100–101
studies of, 215
Cognitive deficits,
52–55, 54b
Cognitive fatigue
measurement of, 38
in postpolio
syndrome, 115
Complete blood cell
count, 86t
Corticotrophin-releasing
factor, 63
Cortisol
chronic fatigue
syndrome–related
reductions in, 64
description of, 63
exercise effects, 64
reductions in, 64
Covariates
cognitive deficits,
52–55, 54b
depression. *See* Depression
description of, 4–5, 45–46
pain, 48–49
sleep disorders. *See* Sleep
disorders
summary overview of, 54b
Creatine phosphokinase, 86t
Creatinine, 86t
Cytokines, 66, 93, 162

Daytime sleepiness
assessment of, 47f,
47–48, 54b
modafinil for, 102t,
103–104
in Parkinson's disease,
46, 125
Definition
Centers for Disease
Control, 9, 10b,
186, 187b
limited investigations
into, 13
multidimensional view, 12
multiple sclerosis–
associated fatigue, 18,
19t, 95
"normal" vs. abnormal
fatigue, 13
overview of, 24b
physician-specific
differences, 11–12
variations in, 9–10
Depression
cancer-related fatigue
and, 134
chronic illness–related, 50
in chronic obstructive
pulmonary
disease, 200
description of, 49–50
in Parkinson's disease,
50, 127
in systemic lupus
erythematosus,
158–159
treatment of, 51–52, 106

Diagnostic approach
  history-taking. *See*
    History-taking
  physical examination, 80t,
    85–87
  workup. *See* Workup
Dialysis, 66
Dimensional view,
  13–14, 15f
Diurnal variations, 24b
Dopamine agonists,
  125–126
Drug-induced fatigue,
  95–96, 97t
Duration, 13, 14f

Ecological momentary
  assessment, 35
Elderly, 25
Electrolytes, 86t
Endocrine system
  dysfunction, 63–65, 72b
Energy
  conservation strategies for,
    209, 213b–214b
  depletion of, 59–60, 72b
Epidemiology
  age, 25
  gender, 23
  overview of, 24b
  race, 25
  socioeconomic class, 23, 25
Epstein-Barr virus, 188
Epworth Sleepiness Scale, 40,
  47f, 47–48, 81
Erythrocyte sedimentation
  rate, 86t

Erythropoietin, 139, 220t
Examination. *See* Physical
  examination
Excessive daytime sleepiness
  assessment of, 47f,
    47–48, 54b
  modafinil for, 102t,
    103–104
  in Parkinson's disease,
    46, 125
Exercise
  for cancer-related
    fatigue, 140
  for multiple sclerosis–
    associated fatigue,
    98–101, 215, 216b
  for Parkinson's
    disease–associated
    fatigue, 127
  for postpolio-associated
    fatigue, 118
  programs for, 214–215,
    216b–217b
  for systemic lupus
    erythematosus–
    related fatigue, 164b
Expanded disability status
  scale, 92

Family history, 80t, 84
Fatigue
  abnormal, 13–14
  cancer-related. *See*
    Cancer-related fatigue
  disorders associated with,
    3t, 82
  drug-induced, 95–96, 97t

Fatigue—*continued*
  duration of, 13, 14f
  frequency of, 13, 14f
  human immunodeficiency
     virus. *See* Human
     immunodeficiency
     virus
  identification of, 4
  Lyme disease. *See* Lyme
     disease
  mental, 135
  multidimensional view
     of, 12
  multiple sclerosis–
     associated. *See*
     Multiple sclerosis
  "normal," 13
  overview of, 1–2
  Parkinson's disease. *See*
     Parkinson's disease
  physical, 135–136
  physiologic factors, 4
  postoperative. *See*
     Postoperative fatigue
  postpolio syndrome.
     See Postpolio
     syndrome
  subjective nature of, 12–13
  systemic lupus
     erythematosus. *See*
     Systemic lupus
     erythematosus
  terminology associated
     with, 11
  undiagnosed, 17
Fatigue Descriptive Scale, 33
Fatigue Impact Scale, 30

Fatigue Severity Scale, 30–31,
    33–34, 34t, 94,
    97–98, 161f
Fatigue Symptom Inventory,
    33, 138
FDS. *See* Fatigue Descriptive
    Scale
Fibromyalgia, 49, 159, 163
FIS. *See* Fatigue Impact Scale
Fluoxetine, 221t
Force generation tests, 12
Frontal lobe, 61
Fruits, 210b
FSI. *See* Fatigue Symptom
    Inventory
FSS. *See* Fatigue Severity
    Scale
Functional Assessment of
    Cancer Therapy
    Measurement System,
    135, 136t

Gender predilection, 23
Gonadal function, 64–65

HAM-D. *See* Hamilton
    Rating Scale for
    Depression
Hamilton Rating Scale for
    Depression, 40
Hepatitis C, 179
Hepatitis screen, 87t
Herbal remedies, 211b
History-taking
  description of, 79
  elements of, 80t
  family history, 80t, 84

lifestyle history, 83–84
medications, 83
psychological history, 84
Human immunodeficiency
   virus
   antiretroviral therapy for,
      177–178, 181
   fatigue associated with
      anemia and, 179
      antiretroviral therapy
         adherence and,
         177–178, 181
      battle fatigue, 180
      causes of, 178t, 178–180
      contributing factors,
         178t
      description of, 21
      infection replication
         and, 179
      management of,
         180–182
      methylphenidate for,
         181–182
      muscle deconditioning
         and, 179–180
      pemoline for, 181–182,
         219, 220t, 222
      pharmacologic therapies
         for, 181–182
      prevalence of, 177
      sleep disturbances, 180
      summary overview
         of, 183b
   memory impairments
      in, 53
   replication of, 179
   testing for, 83, 86t

Hypothalamic-pituitary-
   adrenal axis
   central nervous system
      dysfunction and,
      68–69
   chronic fatigue syndrome
      and, 188
   cortisol reductions, 72b
   description of, 63–64
   psychological stress
      effects, 71
Hypothalamus, 61
Hysterectomy, 21

Immune system
   chronic fatigue
      syndrome, 66
   dysregulation of, 65–66,
      72b–73b
   multiple sclerosis–
      associated fatigue,
      66–67, 93
   neuroendocrine system
      and, 67
Infections, 21–22
Interferons
   a, 65, 93
   b, 65, 93
   t, 66
   thyroid function effects, 67
Interleukin-2, 65
Interleukin-6, 147
Iron-deficiency anemia, 211b
Iron supplementation, 220t

Legumes, 210b
Lethargy, 148

Lifestyle history, 83–84
Lyme disease
    characteristics of, 169–170
    chronic fatigue syndrome
        and, 172
    description of, 83, 87t, 169
    disseminated, 170
    management of, 174
    outcome of, 171
    post-Lyme syndrome,
        170–172, 173b
    rash caused by, 169–170
    serologic tests, 171–172
    summary overview of, 173b

MAF. See Multidimensional
        Assessment of Fatigue
Measurement
    cognitive fatigue, 38
    ecological momentary
        assessment, 35
    Fatigue Impact Scale, 30
    Fatigue Severity Scale,
        30–31, 33–34, 34t
    Modified Fatigue Impact
        Scale, 30–31
    Multidimensional
        Assessment of
        Fatigue, 32
    Multidimensional Fatigue
        Instrument, 32
    overview of, 29, 39b
    performance-based,
        36–37, 39b
    Profile of Mood States, 33
    self-report scales,
        30–35, 39b

Visual Analog Scale, 30,
        33–35, 38
Medical Outcomes
    Survey Short Form
    36, 33
Medication(s), 95–96, 97t
Medication history, 83
Memory impairments, 53
Mental fatigue, 135
Methylphenidate, 181–182,
    219, 220t–221t
Methylprednisolone,
    151t, 152
MFI. See Multidimensional
        Fatigue Instrument
MFIS. See Modified Fatigue
        Impact Scale
Minnesota Multiphasic
    Personality Inventory, 70
MMPI. See Minnesota
        Multiphasic Personality
        Inventory
Modafinil
    adverse effects of, 102t,
        105–106
    characteristics of, 102t,
        103–104, 107b, 220t
    dosing of, 102t, 104–105
    excessive daytime
        sleepiness managed
        using, 126–127
    indications, 222–223
    studies of, 104–106,
        222–223
Modified Fatigue Impact
    Scale, 30–31
Mood, 52–53

MS Council for Clinical
  Practice Guidelines,
  94–95
MS-FS. *See* MS-Specific
  Fatigue Scale
MS-Specific Fatigue
  Scale, 33, 98
Multidimensional Assessment
  of Fatigue, 32
Multidimensional Fatigue
  Instrument, 32
Multidimensional view
  definition of, 12
  measurement scales, 32–33
Multiple sclerosis
  cognitive deficits in, 53
  depression in, 50–52
  fatigue associated with
    assessment of, 97–98
    central conduction
      block and, 94
    cerebral metabolism
      studies, 93–94
    characteristics of, 95
    contributing factors,
      95, 96t
    definition of, 18, 19t, 95
    depression and, 50–51
    description of, 2, 91
    diagnosis of,
      94–98, 107b
    etiology of, 18
    immune system factors,
      66–67, 93
    measurement scales
      for, 97–98
    medication-induced, 95

pathogenesis, 92–94
pathophysiology of, 61
perceived level of,
  94, 96
prevalence of, 17, 91
quality of life effects, 91
studies of, 14
summary overview of,
  107b
symptoms of, 96
treatment of
  amantadine, 101–103,
    102t, 107b,
    219, 220t
  cognitive behavioral
    interventions,
    100–101
  exercise, 98–101, 216b
  modafinil. *See*
    Modafinil
  nonpharmacologic,
    98–101
  pemoline, 102t, 103
  pharmacologic,
    101–106
  summary, 107b
symptoms of, 17, 18t
Muscle relaxants, 126

Natural killer cells, 67
Neurally mediated
  hypotension, 68
Neuroendocrine axis, 61–62
Neurologic examination, 85
Neuromuscular factors,
  62–63
Neurotransmitters, 94

Nutrition
    fatigue managed by, 209,
        210b–212b
    postoperative fatigue
        treated using, 151t

Pain, 48–49, 54b
Parkinson's disease
    depression associated with,
        50, 127
    excessive daytime
        sleepiness associated
        with, 46, 125
    fatigue associated with
        central dopaminergic
            deficiencies and,
            124
        description of, 19,
            48–49, 123–124
        incidence of, 123, 127t
        management of,
            126–127, 127t
        medications that cause,
            125–126
        muscle disuse and
            deconditioning
            and, 124–125
        pathophysiology of, 61,
            124–125
        sleep disorders,
            125, 127t
        summary overview
            of, 128b
    periodic limb movements
        of sleep in, 125
    restless legs syndrome
        in, 125

Pathologic fatigue, 81
Pathophysiology
    autonomic nervous system,
        68–69, 73b
    central nervous system
        disorders, 60–62, 72b
    endocrine system
        dysfunction,
        63–65, 72b
    immunologic factors,
        65–68, 72b–73b
    medications, 95–96, 97t
    multiple sclerosis–
        associated fatigue, 61
    neuromuscular factors,
        62–63
    overview of, 59–60
    psychological factors,
        69–71, 73b
    serotonergic pathways, 61
    summary overview of,
        71–74, 72b–73b
Pemoline, 102t, 103, 181–182,
    219, 220t, 222
Performance-based measure-
    ment, 36–37, 39b
Periodic limb movements of
    sleep, 125
Peripheral fatigue, 62
Physical examination, 80t,
    85–87
Physicians, 11
Physiologic factors, 4
Piper Fatigue Scale, 139, 182
Polysomnography, 46
POMS. *See* Profile of Mood
    States

Populations
  general, 15–16
  medical, 17–25
Post-Lyme syndrome, 22,
    170–172, 173b
Postoperative fatigue
  in cancer patients, 137
  after cardiac surgery, 149
  contributors to, 151t
  covariates of, 145–146
  duration of, 149
  "fast track" surgery to
      prevent, 152–153
  after gynecologic surgery,
      148–149
  interleukin-6 and, 147
  invasiveness of surgery
      and, 153
  malnutrition and, 148
  management of, 149–153,
      150b–151b
  methylprednisolone
      prophylaxis, 151t, 152
  morbidity and, 146f
  muscle disuse and, 147–148
  nutritional strategies for,
      151t
  overview of, 145–146
  perioperative steroids and,
      151t
  physiologic causes of, 147
  psychological contributors,
      147
  radiation therapy and, 148
  recovery effects, 146, 146f
  sleep loss and, 146–147
  tryptophan and, 147

Postpolio syndrome
  chronic fatigue syndrome
      and, 115–116
  definition of, 113
  fatigue associated with
    acute polio and,
        116–117
    affected populations,
        116–117
    amantadine for,
        118–120,
        119b–120b
    brain findings, 114–115
    bromocriptine for,
        118, 119b
    causes of, 114–117
    cognitive fatigue, 115
    description of, 20
    emotional stress, 115
    energy conservation
        techniques for, 118
    incidence of, 113
    management of,
        117–119
    muscle strengthening
        for, 118
    peripheral muscular
        fatigue, 115
    predictive factors, 116
    psychological
        correlates, 116
    severity of, 117
    sleep disorders, 114–115
    summary overview of,
        119b, 120
  muscle tiredness, 20
  prevalence of, 113

Postviral fatigue, 71
Prevalence
cancer-related fatigue, 20t
fatigue in general
population, 16
multiple sclerosis–
associated fatigue,
17, 91
statistics regarding, 2
Primary care populations,
16, 24b
Profile of Mood States, 33, 215
Protriptyline, 221t
Psychological factors
chronic fatigue
syndrome, 189
description of, 69–71
postoperative fatigue, 147
Psychological history, 84
Psychological treatment
cognitive behavioral
therapy. *See* Cognitive
behavioral therapy
description of, 215, 218
Psychosocial factors, 52
Purified protein derivative, 87t

Quality of life effects, 13–14,
132–133, 159

Race, 25
Radiation therapy
cancer-related fatigue
caused by, 135
lethargy secondary to, 148
postoperative fatigue
caused by, 148

Radiographs, 86t
Restless legs syndrome,
125–126
Rheumatologic
assessments, 85

Selective serotonin reuptake
inhibitors, 223–224
Self-reporting measurement
scales
for fatigue, 30–35, 39b
limitations of, 34–35
for multiple sclerosis–
associated fatigue, 98
for pain, 49
Serotonergic pathways, 61
Serum glutamic oxaloacetic
transaminase, 86t
Serum glutamic pyruvic
transaminase, 86t
Sexual abuse, 190
SLE Disease Activity
Index, 162
Sleep
assessment of, 83
movements during,
114–115
nighttime patterns of, 83
postoperative loss of,
146–147
schedule for, 213b
Sleep disorders. *See also*
Daytime sleepiness
in chronic obstructive
pulmonary disease,
200–201
description of, 46–48, 54b

in human
    immunodeficiency
    virus, 180
  in Parkinson's disease, 125
  periodic limb movements
    of sleep, 125
  polysomnography
    evaluations, 46
  in postpolio syndrome,
    114–115
  restless legs syndrome,
    125–126
  in systemic lupus
    erythematosus,
    158, 164b
Sleepiness. *See* Daytime
    sleepiness
Smoking, 83
Social effects, 2
Socioeconomic class, 23, 25
Somatization disorder, 69,
    189–190
Specialists, 11
Stress
  hypothalamic-pituitary-
    adrenal axis effects, 71
  methylprednisolone
    prophylaxis for,
    151t, 152
  postpolio syndrome–
    related fatigue
    secondary to, 115
Supplements, 211b
Symptoms
  Centers for Disease Control
    classification of, 10b
  description of, 45

list of, 12
Systemic Lupus Activity
    Measure, 162
Systemic lupus
    erythematosus
  definition of, 157
  depression associated
    with, 51
  fatigue associated with
    affective disorders,
      158, 164b
    causes of, 157–161
    contributing factors, 158
    depression and, 158–159
    description of, 19–20
    disease activity and, 159,
      160f, 162–163
    disease exacerbations
      and, 158
    incidence of, 157
    level of, 161
    management of,
      163–165
    mood disorders,
      158–159
    physical functioning
      and, 159
    proinflammatory
      cytokines and, 162
    quality of life
      effects, 159
    racial predilection,
      161, 161f
    sleep disorders, 46,
      158, 164b
    summary overview of,
      164b, 165

Systemic lupus erythematosus—*continued*
  fibromyalgia and, 159
  sleep disorders associated with, 46, 158, 164b
  symptoms of, 157

Testosterone replacement therapy, 221t
Thyroiditis, 67
Thyroid-stimulating hormone, 86t
Tizanidine, 95
T lymphocytes, 66
Tobacco, 211b
Total bilirubin, 86t
Treatment
  cognitive behavioral therapy. *See* Cognitive behavioral therapy
  energy conservation, 209, 213b–214b
  exercise programs, 214–215, 216b–217b
  family education regarding, 208–209
  nutrition/dietary interventions, 209, 210b–212b
  overview of, 207–208
  patient education regarding, 208
  pharmacologic, 218–224
  psychological interventions, 215, 218
  summary overview of, 224
Tryptophan, 147
Tumor necrosis factor-a, 66

Urinalysis, 86t

Vegetables, 210b
Verbal learning, 37f, 38
Visual Analog Scale, 30, 34–35, 40, 49

Water, 210b
Women, 23
Workup
  elements of, 80t–81t
  family history, 80t, 84
  history-taking, 79–84
  laboratory tests, 85–87
  overview of, 79
  physical examination, 80t, 85–87